Breaking the Diet Habit

BREAKING THE DIET HABIT

The Natural Weight Alternative

JANET POLIVY

C. PETER HERMAN

Basic Books, Inc., Publishers   New York

For Stanley Schachter,

who taught us how to ask the questions;

and for our patients, fat and thin,

who showed us the need for new answers.

Library of Congress Cataloging in Publication Data

Polivy, Janet.
  Breaking the diet habit.

  Bibliography: p. 212.
  Includes index.
  1. Reducing—Psychological aspects.
2. Reducing—Social aspects. 3. Obesity—Social
aspects. 4. Health behavior. I. Herman,
C. Peter, 1946–   II. Title.
RM222.2.P59 1983   613.2'5'019   82-72403
ISBN 0-465-00754-6

Contents

Acknowledgments   *vii*

Introduction   *3*

CHAPTER 1
Compulsion and Choice   *12*

CHAPTER 2
The Defense of Natural Weight   *27*

CHAPTER 3
Overweight, Overeating, and Health   *54*

CHAPTER 4
Dangers of Dieting   *75*

CHAPTER 5
Narcissus and Sisyphus—Social and Personal
Aspects of Dieting   *100*

v

Contents

CHAPTER 6
Effects of Dieting on Eating 129

CHAPTER 7
Correlates or Side Effects of Dieting 156

CHAPTER 8
Results of Not Accepting Oneself—Compulsive
Eating or Starving 168

CHAPTER 9
Natural Eating and Dieting 190

References 212

Index 223

Acknowledgments

AS USUAL, it is hard to know how to share the credit adequately. Many of the ideas in this book were suggested, sometimes unwittingly, by our friends and colleagues; partitioning their contributions accurately is impossible. The following are some of the people who have helped us: our colleagues in psychology at the University of Toronto, particularly the ever critical "lunch group," with special mention to Tony Doob, Jonathan Freedman, and Nicholas Mrosovsky; our colleagues on the "eating disorders" unit at the Clarke Institute of Psychiatry, especially Paul Garfinkel and David Garner; our medical school colleagues, Errol Marliss and Dan Roncari; our more distant colleagues, Dick Bootzin at Northwestern, Dick Nisbett at Michigan, and Susan and Wayne Wooley at Cincinnati, who provided both ideas and support; and our students, in Toronto and Illinois, who did so much of the experimental

Acknowledgments

work, and who fulfilled their obligation to listen to and consider our crazier ideas.

This book would never have appeared—and certainly not with its current focus—had it not been for the people at Basic Books, Margie Ruddick and Jane Isay, the true clinical master in this enterprise. Ron Lieberman saved us from our other publishing opportunities. Maureen Patchett made sure that if we missed a deadline it was our own fault.

In addition, we must thank Lisa Cesia, who provided us with all the distractions that aspiring authors could hope for—and more. We also thank our long-suffering spouses, who put up with our laziness, perfectionism, crankiness, and preference for doing things our own way. Worry is never wasted.

JP, CPH
Toronto, 1982

Breaking the Diet Habit

Introduction

THIS is a book about eating, or rather, not eating. More specifically, it concerns *trying* not to eat—that is, dieting. What are the causes of dieting? And what are its effects?

For decades now, overweight or obesity has been viewed as the problem. When we started our careers as research and clinical psychologists, we (and just about everyone else) took it for granted that overweight was a serious problem, on medical, social, and personal grounds, and that finding solutions to this problem was a worthwhile ambition. We also took it for granted that most cases of overweight were caused by overeating, and that if we could block or reverse the causes of overeating, then weight would subside to a normal level. Most theories of obesity postulated some defect in the individual as responsible for the overeating. Perhaps the overeater was confusing emotional needs with hunger, and overeating in an attempt to fill a poorly identified need. Perhaps he or she overate *in order to* get fat, because of the symbolic meanings of fatness, meanings which might play a neurotically useful role in his or her life. Perhaps the overeater was the victim of a "food addiction," in which the more food one ate, the more one needed. Or perhaps the overeater suffered from a psychosensory aberration in which eating was controlled, not by nutritional requirements, but by the sensory properties of food itself, or by the circumstances surrounding eating, or by social pressures. In any case, the problem was overeating and the solution was to eat less. The only question was how to eat less.

The "how to" question was not a simple one. For one thing, the answer was generally presumed to depend on the original defect, in which case it might require basic research into the nature of that defect. Behavior therapists, however, argued that you didn't have to know the cause of a behavioral problem in order to treat it effectively. We can cure a headache with aspirin, after all, even though we don't know the cause of the headache—or, for that matter, how aspirin works. Nonetheless, attempts to retrain or recondition faulty eating habits— to make them more closely resemble the eating habits of people who aren't fat and who don't overeat—proved disappointing. Maybe overweight wasn't just a behavioral problem—a matter of bad eating habits. In any case, we ourselves began from the position that understanding the causes of the problem was a prerequisite for finding satisfactory solutions.

We started out in the tradition begun by Professor Stanley Schachter, of Columbia University. He was pushing the notion that fat people suffered from a defect in the regulation of their eating—namely, a tendency to be controlled by "extraneous" stimuli (such as the taste and texture of food and the circum-

stances surrounding eating) to the exclusion of calorically relevant stimuli (i.e., those that bear on the issues of hunger,
satiety, and caloric requirements). Of course, everybody is sensitive to such supposedly extraneous factors to some extent, but
fat people seemed to be totally dominated by them. It was easy
to construct a scenario in which a person controlled by "external" factors might overeat and become fat. The question, then,
was "Why do some people have this defect?"—as well as
"What can we do about it?" The details of this scientific
question will occupy us later in this book. For us, personally,
the single most important insight—one provided by
Schachter's former student, Professor Richard Nisbett, of the
University of Michigan—was that the defect might in fact be
caused by dieting. Nisbett didn't say this in so many words, but
he came close. We added a couple of extensions to his basic
thesis and formalized the proposition that the problem with fat
people is that they diet.

At first, we were excited simply by the new ways of thinking
that this thesis required and by the observations it led us to:
for instance, on examination it turned out that many of the
bizarre eating practices (and other strange behaviors, apparently unrelated to eating) that fat people exhibited were also
exhibited by normal weight dieters. By the same token, the few
fat people we could find who didn't diet didn't show the typical
"fat" behavior profile. Thus, on the basis of these observations,
we gradually came around—despite having been raised in the
same diet culture as everyone else—to the view that the problem wasn't fatness, it was dieting.

Coming around to this view is not all that easy. After all, it's
not as if we can blame the problem of fatness on dieting.
Dieting is a *response* to the problem. Maybe dieting causes a

few problems of its own; we're all willing to entertain that possibility. But if dieting disappeared entirely, we'd still have fatness, right?

Well, yes. But consider fatness. Why, exactly, is it a problem? We tried our best to eliminate preconceptions about fatness, all the old clichés. We began to examine the "problem" of obesity freshly, without assuming that it *was* a problem. We began to compare the negative aspects of fatness to the negative aspects of dieting. The one cliché that seemed to be supported, we found, was that the cure was often worse than the disease. Looked at objectively, fatness seems to be no worse (and in some ways better) than the pursuit of thinness. The pros and cons will require some space to develop—as well as some background—but this book begins with our questioning the relation of the "problem" to the "solution."

Just on the basis of the research—our own and others'—we convinced ourselves that dieting caused at least as many problems as it solved. The proposal that some people would be better off just staying fat seemed more and more judicious. Clinical work took us yet a step further. For one thing, exposure to anorexia nervosa—which "took off" as a cultural/medical phenomenon in the 1970s—made the dangers of dieting all too apparent. In the case of anorexia nervosa, there was no question that the cure (dieting) was a worse disease than the disease (overweight) itself.

From less dramatic clinical cases of people with weight problems, as well, it gradually dawned on us that we might be on to something more profound than a cultural misjudgment of the relative risks and benefits of overweight and dieting. We had come to accept that the problem of overweight might be less troublesome than the solution of dieting. A more difficult notion that had eventually forced its way into our analysis was that dieting may actually *cause* overeating and overweight. The perspective had turned 180 degrees. The explication of this difficult and (to us traditionalists) paradoxical notion will likewise be delayed until we can develop it properly in the context of the book. For the present, it is sufficient to note that by the time we got to this stage in our thinking, the need for this book was already becoming apparent.

For close to 10 years, we had been studying dieting and its effects in the laboratory, as research psychologists. Outside the lab, we had been listening to patients and friends bemoan their weight problems—and the equally depressing "solutions" that they had applied to these problems. Further, we had been exposed to the barrage of articles, programs, and best-selling books conveying the latest "scientific" information on how to achieve "effective, painless, and rapid" weight loss. Our exposure, professional and personal, to the facts, fictions, and fantasies of weight reduction disturbed and frustrated us. We saw the "diet culture" in which we live cause a great deal of suffering for our friends and, especially, for our patients. We found this disturbing; yet, attempting to convince normally sensible people to apply the same degree of intelligence to their eating and dieting practices as they do to the selection of a stereo set or even a pair of gloves is often like trying to reason with a lemming in full flight. What is particularly frustrating is that the premises of this "diet culture," its basic assumptions, are rarely if ever examined in a thoughtful way. The purpose of this book is to provide such an examination. If we can expose some of the flaws in the assumptions underlying the "diet culture," then perhaps the reader will begin to question those assumptions. And, if we can foster a critical attitude, then perhaps some of the suffering will abate.

This is no ordinary diet book, obviously. We are not especially concerned with extolling the virtues of our "quick weight loss" plan. (Actually, we do have some suggestions about how some people may lose weight—and more easily than by dieting. But these suggestions must come later, in context.) We are concerned primarily with questioning the purposes and effects of dieting. Do the reasons dieters give for dieting correspond to what they get? If not, why does dieting persist?

Dieting has reached the status of an obsession in our society. Like other obsessions, this one is characterized by the victims' being compelled to worry about it and to act (compulsively) in accordance with its dictates. People, it seems, don't choose to diet; they feel they must. We hope to restore some choice to the matter, by providing pros and cons. When people are faced with only pros, what choice do they have? Choice, of course, can be confusing; it suggests the possibility of being wrong, which might make dieters uncomfortable. But they are uncomfortable now. And many of them are already wrong, in choosing an option in which the cons outweigh the pros. The only difference is that they don't realize that they are pursuing a poor option. They don't even realize that they had a choice. The cons have been hidden; the pros, glorified. The result is a delusion—partly self-imposed, partly imposed by the culture —in which it often seems (correctly) that the harder one fights, the further one is from victory.

In self-help books, the focus has been exclusively on "technique"; the ultimate goals—weight loss, slimness, attractiveness, health, and happiness—have been taken for granted. Also taken for granted is the notion that these various goals all "go together," that one is buying a "package" of self-improvement. As we shall see, there is an accumulating store of research that indicates that neither health, nor happiness, nor attractiveness, nor even slimness necessarily follows from dieting. In fact, it is becoming increasingly apparent that, for many of us, these various goals may be directly incompatible. Weight loss may threaten health; slimness may be achieved only at the cost of psychological well-being. Although such incompatibility of goals may not pertain to all of us, it does apply to many; and, to the extent that it does apply, it necessitates some hard choices. It may well be that you can't eat your cake and have it too; but it may also be the case that you *must* eat at least some of your cake if you are to have some of the other things you want out of life. In any case, choices must be (consciously) made.

In chapter 1, we point out—and criticize—the fatalistic attitude of most dieters; whether they are overweight or not, whether dieting will achieve their ultimate goals or not, they feel compelled to diet and, correspondingly, feel guilty if they don't diet, or if they "cheat." We hope to make it apparent that there is a choice, that there must be a choice, and that an active decision about dieting is both possible and desirable.

Chapter 2 presents in detail the basis for the concept of "natural weight." Physiologically, we operate so as to "defend" our body weight at a particular level, or at least within a certain range. The physiological defense of "natural weight," as one might imagine, has monumental implications for the dieter, and provides the first hint that attempts to reduce one's weight substantially may prove to be problematic (or impossible).

Following this explanation of the theoretical underpinnings and physiological evidence for a natural level of body weight, we survey the various reasons normally offered as justifications for dieting—which is to say, for challenging one's natural weight. In chapter 3, we examine one of the most powerful reasons for dieting—the medical case against overweight. As we shall see, this case is much shakier than we have been led to believe. Next, in chapter 4, we look at the obverse case, the medical case for slimness. Again, we shall encounter some data that may lead us to question our assumptions about the relation of weight loss to health.

Chapter 5 examines a different sort of reason for dieting—actually, a host of reasons. This chapter takes a close look at the current social pressures toward slimness, based on stereotypes of attractiveness. Also, we shall examine the implicit personality correlates of fatness and thinness, and the implications of one's physique for attributions regarding one's character and for one's self-esteem.

In chapter 6, we present psychological research evidence, including our own, on the aberrant eating patterns associated with dieting. In chapter 7, we extend our examination of the correlates of dieting to aspects of behavior normally considered to be unrelated to eating. In both chapters, we emphasize the disturbing and generally unacknowledged consequences of dieting.

In chapter 8, we examine the all-too-frequent results of not accepting oneself—compulsive binge eating and/or self-starvation (anorexia nervosa)—and analyze such behaviors in terms of the foregoing survey of "normal" eating and dieting. Finally, chapter 9 is a review and integration of all the material we present in the book, which we hope will help the reader make an informed choice about the alternatives involved in dieting. Here we present our "Natural Weight Undiet" for those who decide that dieting is not the answer for them.

Our main goal in this book is to raise some important questions for the reader. The research findings we present pose a series of challenges to prevailing views; they also suggest some alternatives. Obviously, we cannot make decisions for particular individuals; only they can evaluate the personal costs and benefits involved in pursuing (or not pursuing) slimness. But we can invite the reader to think through, more clearly and more systematically, the choices one must make—about whether to diet, how to diet, how much to diet, and so on. Our ultimate goal is to furnish the basis for sensible choices.

CHAPTER 1

Compulsion and Choice

I don't know where to begin, doctor. Here in your office I just want to sit and cry and cry. I hate myself so much. I diet so well all day—I eat next to nothing. I usually can even get through dinner all right. But then the evening stretches out ahead of me and it seems that all I can ever think about is food. Watching TV makes me think of food—all those commercials! Reading doesn't work. I can't concentrate. I feel as if food—eating or not eating —dominates my whole life. It seems as if everything I eat turns to fat. If I take a deep breath in a bakery, I gain a pound. My whole life is a struggle to control my weight, but I never get thin. It's as if my own body were plotting against me. I look so terrible. I have to diet constantly just to look like this, and I've never been able to get down as low as I should. I never look like those fashion magazines. I'm afraid that I never will. It's so unfair. My brother eats like a pig and I'm the one who gets fat. He never gives a moment's thought to his weight and stays slim. And I have to starve myself all the time just to look halfway decent. And most of the time, I'm not even halfway decent. I have to prepare myself psychologically before I look in a mirror. If I catch a glimpse of myself accidentally in a store window or a mirror or something, it can be a terrible shock. It doesn't seem like me. It doesn't even really seem like a person. All I see are hips and stomach. And it's as if they're growing—mushrooming—while I look. They seem so enormous, even though I know that they're not, really. I just feel like a big fat worthless blob. Why do I have to suffer like this all the time?

Why indeed? What, exactly, is the justification for this pain, for the all-consuming effort not to consume? Much of the suffering that our hypothetical dieter describes—first, the deprivation; then, the frustrating focus on food, which stems from the deprivation and which makes the sense of deprivation worse; then, the failures, which only increase the need for further deprivation—is self-inflicted. This woman eats less because she wants to. She diets.

Listening to her description, of course, we would never get the impression that dieting is something that she herself decided to do. She makes it seem as if dieting were a penance imposed on her by the outside world. But isn't it the case that dieting is something that she chose to do? Whether or not to diet is a matter of choice, isn't it? Or is it?

Whether dieting is the sort of thing one can choose depends —like most choices—on alternatives. If there is some other option, then the dieter has a choice about dieting. If not, then the dieter is in fact forced to diet. Certainly, the pitiful monologue above leads us to believe that for this woman there is no option. Her dieting isn't very successful, but it is the only chance she has. Without it, she would be even worse off—fatter, uglier, more miserable. *That's* the alternative. And for most of us, that's no alternative at all.

✳Yet there have been times and places—in fact, there still are —where overweight didn't necessarily mean "ugly" or "psychologically miserable." In such remote times and places, in fact, the word "overweight" might be somewhat anomalous; "underweight" was more likely to be the problem. But although it is refreshing, perhaps, to think of our excess body fat as desirable rather than problematic, the fact remains that for most of us, overweight is not acceptable.✳ Some of us may tolerate it, but we never welcome it. Only our grandmothers can seriously regard us as "too skinny." We live in a society that reveres slimness. Slimness is beauty. Slimness is happiness. Slimness is health. (Or, at least, so it appears to those of us who aren't decidedly slim.)

Given such a powerful tendency in our culture to value slimness, it is hard to see how the dieter has much of a choice. The value of slimness is never questioned; and as long as that value reigns supreme, not striving toward it is considered not only unhealthy and stupid, but even immoral. When beauty, health, and happiness are all available through successful dieting, who wouldn't choose such a course?

Hence, our dieter's desperation at being forced to battle constantly against a gluttonous, mutinous body in order to achieve what she should (i.e., slenderness) probably reflects a struggle that she did not actively decide to undertake. She's aware that she's fighting. And she's aware that there are various weapons against fat available to her, so that she can actively choose her arsenal. But did she choose to fight in the war itself? —not likely. That's a fact of life one must accept. The individual who surrenders—or who even fails to fight as vigorously as possible—is a deserter, a coward, a traitor . . . a fat person.

We all recognize that our society puts an esthetic premium on thinness; what is less obvious is the moral premium. As we shall see in chapter 5, overweight people are regarded as physically less attractive than average. But this stereotype—this judgment based solely on appearance—extends also to the overweight individual's personality and character. Society tends to make a moral judgment against those who fail to achieve slimness. It does not seem to matter that some start out slimmer than others, nor that some really do have more trouble losing weight. The slim person is seen as more in control, more concerned, more willing to make sacrifices for what is right. In short, the slim person is viewed as morally superior.

Although this judgment is usually implicit, most of the time it isn't all that far from the surface. How many people have you heard referred to as "thin slobs"? Because the assumptions underlying the stereotype—the assumptions that overweight is a form of moral, medical, and esthetic perversity—are so widely held and rarely challenged, we tend to accept them without scrutiny.

Think for a minute about your own attitudes. You may feel yourself to be more sophisticated than most people, and less subject to prejudice. But do you honestly believe that overweight people are as physically attractive as normal weight or slim people? How do the overweight compare with others on traits like sloppiness or self-control? Negative attitudes about overweight, clearly, are widespread. In fact, they appear, as pervasively as anywhere else, among overweight people themselves. Like members of other minorities, fat people tend to view themselves through the eyes of others—despite the efforts of such consciousness-raising groups as "Fat Is Beautiful." They, too, are convinced that they can't be attractive unless they are thin, or even skinny (and that once they're thin, beauty will follow automatically). It shouldn't be surprising, then, that overweight people feel compelled to change their profiles and shrink themselves down to normal—or better, below normal. To this social pressure to be thin add the sermons from doctors and public health agencies about the potentially fatal health hazards of overweight, and you have a situation in which it is remarkable that there could be any overweight person who is not fully dedicated to dieting or other strategies of weight loss.

Thus, the combination of social and medical pressures to lose weight produces psychological and moral judgments which add salt to the wound of fleshiness. If fat is both unattractive and unhealthy, what sort of person would tolerate it? All are agreed that only the weakest, most self-indulgent, personally irresponsible glutton would put up with disgusting and dangerous fat tissue. Gluttony, you'll remember, was a deadly sin. So the situation boils down to a simple syllogism for the overweight person: Fat is bad; you are fat; therefore, you are bad. Let us go back and listen to our hypothetical dieter again for a minute.

I know that it's just a matter of telling myself that I can do it. But I just die for a doughnut when everyone else has them at coffee break. I'm hungry all the time. I'm even hungry right now. And I don't know how I'll get through tonight without eating something bad. I can just imagine my will power crumbling, and me hating myself afterwards. Oh, doctor, no matter how hard I try, I just never seem to be able to lose this weight and keep it off. And it's so awful never to be able to eat like a normal person. It's as if I have a "condition," like an alcoholic or an addict. I love food, but I don't dare enjoy it. I'm actually afraid of it, because I know that I can't control myself around it. I feel so deprived all the time that if I ever really let myself go, I don't think I'd ever stop. I just seem to go round and round—or rather, up and down. I'm on an elevator and I don't think that I'll ever be able to get off. It's so horrible. Why can't I eat what I want to like everyone else? Why do I have to be so fat?

Could she "get off the elevator"?

If the dieter can be seen as fleeing the stick of fatness—an inappropriate metaphor, perhaps, but one that conveys the various types of punishments (ugliness, disease, lack of self-respect or virtue) involved in overweight—it's also possible to see him or her as pursuing the carrot of thinness—a much more appropriate metaphor. Our carrot-eating dieter is not only escaping vice, but also pursuing virtue. For just as fatness implies badness, so slimness implies goodness. And the dieter's self-esteem, so battered by overweight, can heal itself and even expand as the waistline contracts. Successful dieting, in our society, is a great (and much-acclaimed) accomplishment. And the acclaim one gets from weight loss, like the blame one gets for weight gain (or simply for overweight), comes not only from others but also from oneself. Self-denial and self-control lead to self-esteem, one of our most powerful motivational forces. Self-denial, the refusal of food in the face of temptation, becomes idealized as a statement of superiority, even a way of life. At first, the dieter will exhibit this marvelous capacity for self-control in public, "cheating" only in private. Friends and family see a martyr. How can someone be blamed for overweight when he or she doesn't eat anything? Eventually, of course, the dieter must face the fact that a calorie consumed in the closet doesn't count any less than one consumed in a restaurant. It is necessary to perform for oneself as well as for others. Private guilt is added to public embarrassment. And self-esteem becomes as important as—even more important than—the esteem of others.

The dieter, then, is doubly compelled. On the one hand, there is a negative motivation; the dieter is trying to escape or avoid the negative aspects of overweight, not unlike a rat pressing a bar to escape or avoid electric shock. On the positive side, the dieter is trying for the rewards of slimness, not unlike a rat pressing a bar to obtain a food pellet. These motives are compelling. Do they leave the dieter any choice? (Does the rat have any choice?) When both motives push or pull the dieter in the same direction—toward weight loss—the question of choice is probably best viewed in terms of the intensity or power of the motivational forces. The more powerful the punishments or rewards, the less choice the dieter has. And from the perspective of most dieters—certainly from the perspective of our monologuist—these forces are extremely powerful. Thus choice is virtually negligible.

If all these various pressures toward slimness are compelling, the "choice" should be easy: lose weight. But, as we all know, if the pressures of the mind—our attitudes and beliefs, our knowledge of what is best for us, what will make us happy— are powerful, they are nonetheless not so powerful as to win an easy victory over the enemy: fat. Dieting, the time-honored route to weight loss favored by most would-be reducers, is not an easy thing to do. And actual weight loss is even harder to achieve than dieting, at least in the long run. Despite the rewards for losing and the punishments for not losing—despite the fact that, as we've seen, most overweight people feel that there's no option but to try—the statistics regarding weight loss are abysmal. Various studies of weight loss programs— which reflect the whole range of dieting devices, techniques, and tricks—reveal overwhelmingly that the dropout rates are high (i.e., many people can't or won't even complete the initial "treatment") and the relapse rates (the proportion of people who achieve some or all of the weight loss hoped for only to gain back the weight within a year or two) are even higher. Most dieters, it appears, are on and off diets constantly, their weights fluctuating like the Dow Jones average. As our dieter puts it:

> And it just goes on and on. I lost ten pounds. But then somehow, I couldn't seem to control myself, especially at night. I'd wake up in the middle of the night and promise myself that I'd just have some carrot or celery sticks. And then, before I knew it, I'd be eating bread, cookies, anything fattening I could find. Within a week I had gained back all the weight that I suffered so much to lose. It was as if I had to eat—I didn't even really enjoy it, and afterward I was so ashamed, so guilty. I was back where I started, fat and ugly. Miserable. Now I'm back again, ready to try, determined to resist the temptations. But it's such a struggle, I'm afraid I'll just fail again.

Fat resists. It seems as though it is in the very nature of fat to arrive more easily than depart. No matter that slimness will bring health, happiness, beauty, and a sense of personal worth; our fat asserts its own right to exist. And it defends its "rights" with a primitive but lethal array of weapons. Mostly, if you challenge it, you'll suffer. Weight loss, especially those "last few pounds," tends to bring with it a constant, badgering—even painful—hunger that's almost impossible to avoid giving in to. It's a hunger that's not lightly dismissed or dispelled. Carrots and celery just don't satisfy the sort of hunger that dieters are constantly battling. If you've ever been a dieter, you know that it is precisely the rich, solid foods— steaks, cakes, and shakes—that your body and mind crave, not the crisp "diet" foods that nature obviously intended for rabbits.

And not only does fat resist by imposing the ache of hunger on those who would be slim, but it seems to have a remarkable capacity for survival even in those who successfully undergo the rigors of self-deprivation and hunger. Dieting doesn't always work the way it's "supposed to." Despite the diet doctors' assurances that if you just eat less (and perhaps exercise more) you're bound to lose weight, you know that the fat doesn't detach itself nearly as easily as it attached itself in the first place. Uncle Remus might as well have told us of a Fat Baby as a Tar Baby. So, if we resist attractive—and even not-so-attractive—foods, we suffer hunger and frustration. And then —as if that much suffering weren't enough—we find that our fat just isn't melting away as we'd expect, considering how much suffering we endure. Are our bodies telling us something? Is that fat perhaps serving some biological purpose?

Whatever else they may be telling us, our bodies are pretty convincing about the difficulty of weight loss. The war against fat, though it may be a "just" war, even a righteous war, won't be a walkover, a Six Day War, or even a Six Month War (sometimes it feels more like a Hundred Years' War). But maybe there's a good reason for our fat to struggle to survive. Maybe our fat actually *does* something for us. In chapter 2, we will present the idea that we all have our own ideal weight, which is set by our bodies, and not by society. For some people, the ideal, or what we'll call their "natural weight," may well be considerably higher than what fashion calls ideal, or even normal. Trying to get from one's "natural weight" down to the societal ideal may involve a struggle against one's own physiology, which strives to maintain that higher weight.

Not only is this struggle difficult, it is also dangerous. First, as we shall see, there is the danger posed by the very stress involved in fighting against one's natural, constitutional inclinations; this is the direct stress of dieting. Next, there is the indirect danger posed by a necessary corollary of dieting, that is, the unlinking of eating from its natural regulatory influences, hunger and satiety. Dieting demands that hunger be to some extent ignored. Eventually, the dieter may lose altogether the ability to eat naturally, on the basis of hunger and satiety cues. The end result, paradoxically, may be periodic bouts of overeating or even binge eating, which may drive the dieter's weight above what it might have been had he or she not begun to diet in the first place. Finally, there is the danger of a complete break between one's internal guidelines or fundamental motivations, on the one hand, and one's behavior, on the other. Many dieters simply get lost. They embarked on a program of weight loss in the interest of health, happiness, and beauty. They are, for the most part, not succeeding. Rather than question the assumptions underlying the program, however, they end up questioning themselves, wondering where they have gone wrong, and where to go next. Indeed, for some it may be that the lack of self-direction is actually the *cause* of dieting; dieting may be a "purpose" for those who have no other clear goals.

For the present, let us simply reiterate one of our earlier questions: Why are we fighting? Sure, we're fighting in order to lose weight; but why? What is the end toward which weight loss is the means? Health? Beauty? Happiness? All of these? Isn't it obvious?

As psychologists, we believe that it's more "obvious" than it should be. In other words, most of us tend to take for granted the ultimate goals; we consider them as plain as the fat on our hips. And we consider it to be obvious that slimness is equivalent to health, happiness, and attractiveness. But what if weight loss isn't the magic key to success in all these respects? What if even a diligent weight loser fails to achieve these ultimate goals? Earlier we argued that it was the very strength of these lures that made the overweight person feel compelled to diet. But what if these rewards were not really waiting on the other side of successful weight loss? What if there were no guarantee that slimness would provide one with *any* of these rewards? In this book, we hope to show that the guarantee is in fact very questionable. And, as a consequence, we want people to analyze, very clearly, what they stand to gain from weight loss or dieting. For some, weight loss may indeed be the obvious solution to all of life's problems. But, for most, the issue is much more complicated. Whether or not weight loss, even if successful, will deliver on its promises ought to be considered an open question. In short, weight loss may be only one pathway to health, beauty, and happiness; and it may not be the best one. We want people to think in terms of alternatives. And, once they have alternatives, they have regained the power to exert choice. They may well decide to fight—but they'll be fighting as volunteers, not as draftees.

The fact is that in our culture most dieters are draftees. Their service is compulsory, and they are in for the duration. For some, the external pressures to diet outweigh the internal pressures: how they appear to others is more important, ultimately, than how they appear to themselves. On a desert island —given enough coconuts and mangoes—these people might well develop the rounded physiques of South Sea islander kings. But not in the land of *Vogue!* For others, of course, the pressures have become internalized. The need to diet seems to emanate from within, to be part of one's self, one's identity, rather than simply something imposed by the fashion industry.

Such people, if they found themselves alone on the desert island, would be on the lookout for skimmed coconut milk. They would search the island not for shelter, and certainly not for food, but for a reliable bathroom scale, and possibly for a full-length mirror. The most serious—indeed, pathological— form of this internalized compulsion to diet appears in the increasingly prevalent "disease" of anorexia nervosa. This syndrome is characterized by a virtual terror of fatness, to the point where sufferers will often refuse to eat, even if it means starvation. Here, obviously, we are dealing with a compulsion to diet that exceeds the normal societal pressures. Indeed, the anorexic patient, with her skeletal physique and her flirtation with death, brings on herself a barrage of pressures to *not* diet. These eat-for-life pressures, though, are fundamentally external, and not really meaningful to the patient. She has learned her lesson too well. She must continue to flee fatness—and fatness, for these patients, occurs at a level that most of us would consider absurdly low. For the anorexic, high double-digit weights can represent danger, and triple digits can seem like disaster.

Most dieters, of course, don't appear to be as driven as the anorexic girls who regularly employ the dangerous practice of self-induced vomiting as a weight control device. Nonetheless, the degree of compulsion evident in dieters is often astounding. A quick look at the instruments of torture endured by dieters, at the agonies they inflict on themselves, will convince any onlooker that weight loss is of paramount concern to millions. Eat all the bananas you want—but nothing else. Eat anything you want—but nothing with carbohydrates. Eat substances like predigested protein, designed to fool your body into weight loss. Or eat nothing at all. Or try running or cycling or tennis or swimming (at least these sports crazes have some beneficial side effects, along with the principal intended effect—weight loss). How about intestinal bypass surgery, with its mortality rate of up to 10 percent? Or maybe surgical fat removal, or a wire clamping the jaws, or a staple in the ear? What exactly are people prepared to tolerate in search of the Holy Grail of weight loss? Most dieters will tolerate plenty—including the financial strain of overpriced, overpadded diet books, and foods that cost extra because the sugar has been removed (after having been added by the same manufacturer).

What we'll put up with, of course, depends on what we expect to get out of our pain and suffering. We expect to get a lot out of weight loss. But are these expectations justified? Is the pot at the end of the diet rainbow really filled with gold? Or is it fool's gold? Or do we just end up with an empty pot? If the rainbow were a pleasant route to travel, then perhaps it wouldn't matter so much. But nobody—or at least a very small proportion of dieters—has ever claimed that dieting itself is much fun. It's the payoff that counts.

In later chapters, we shall examine the reasons why people diet. What are the payoffs they expect? And, more important, what can they realistically expect? We shall discover that many of the rewards that dieters hope (and definitely plan) to receive after weight loss just aren't there. And by the same token, many of the consequences—the payoffs—of dieting are entirely unexpected and often quite unwelcome. Most people, including the social, medical, and psychiatric establishments urging dieters to lose more and more, are unaware of the unwelcome side effects that may accompany dieting. Even those who are in a position to know that dieting doesn't always work the way it's supposed to—for example, doctors and psychiatrists—tend to blame the victim (the dieter) or idiosyncratic factors. Thus, this emphasis on benefits and deemphasis on costs probably accounts for why so many people try dieting —and why so many are surprised and disappointed at the long-term results. We are disturbed by this one-sidedness in the public's view of dieting; we consider this view seriously unbalanced.

As we have stated, this book is an attempt to redress the balance. We hope to indicate, in a no nonsense way, what the effects of dieting really are. Some aspects are pleasurable, some are painful. Some are worthwhile, others are almost the opposite of what the dieter had in mind. The point of our survey is to provide people with a choice, to stimulate them to think through their own reasons for dieting, and to help them examine not only why they are dieting, but also what they can expect to get from weight loss. The answers will be different for each person. In the area of dieting and weight loss, as in other areas, we're not all the same. So each person must be concerned with what's best for himself or herself, not what's best for "people in general." In short, one must assert one's independence, and decide for oneself, regardless of how others behave.

One major problem with making an informed choice is that it means you must be informed. We shall present, as clearly as we can, the evidence regarding the pluses and minuses of dieting. But there's no getting around the fact that some pieces of evidence are more reliable than are others. Some facts have been established; other "facts" are little more than speculation. Most diet books don't bother distinguishing between these two sorts of facts, between the oases and the mirages that appear in the desert of our ignorance. It is frustrating to have to settle for uncertainty; but in some areas of weight loss research— ironically, perhaps, mainly in the areas concerned with "hard" science, physiology and medicine—the evidence just isn't decisive. Difficult as it may be, then, we shall encourage you to suspend judgment on some issues.

Although some issues—for example, whether it is always healthier to lose "excess" weight—are far from settled, many others are in fact quite clear, once we think about them and study the evidence. What isn't clear, though, is whether a particular reason for dieting will be worth it *for a particular individual*. We can present evidence, pro and con. If one diets, such-and-such effect will likely be the result, but there may also be some other effects one might not have anticipated. Many of the consequences of dieting are not generally known. Many that are known conflict with our normal reverence for dieting as an exalted way of life. The reader of this book may develop some new perspectives on dieting. Some old ideas may be shaken.

What will be the result? We can't say, precisely. But our purpose isn't to change behavior. We want simply to make people challenge themselves, to reexamine the "wisdom" they have accepted, bit by bit, over the years. What bothers us is that dieters are so *compelled*, so driven. They don't get a chance to choose. They've never had an option. By presenting the issues freshly, and in a balanced way, we hope to renew the possibility of choice for them, to open up some options. We care much less about the particular choice that individuals make than about their making a choice. If you're going to suffer, after all, isn't it preferable to know why?

CHAPTER 2

The Defense of Natural Weight

IN MINNESOTA, toward the end of World War II, a group of conscientious objectors agreed to participate in a research project as their contribution to the war effort. The devastations of war on civilians and soldiers alike had prompted researchers to examine the effects of long-term food deprivation, semistarvation, and weight loss. What *are* the effects of long-term hunger?

The initial objective was for the research subjects to lose about a quarter of their original body weight. Weight loss was virtually ensured by the provision of an uninspired (though adequately nutritious) limited calorie diet. At first, losing weight was not especially difficult for most of the men. They continued with their normal activities—saw their girlfriends, read, played cards, exercised as usual, and so on—but simply cut down on their caloric intake. Fewer calories meant weight loss, as we would expect. However, the process did not continue indefinitely. Even before the subjects reached their weight loss goal—a goal, mind you, that was not a serious threat to their physical well-being—the same low caloric intake that had produced a decline in weight no longer worked. Some men had to decrease their food intake even further; others stopped losing altogether. Finally, the men's behavior in general began to change—and for the worse. As they struggled to reach their goals, they began to fight with their girlfriends (or ex-girlfriends!) or were no longer interested in seeing them or in any normal sexual activity; they lost their ability to concentrate on books and became easily distractible; their emotions flared so that they were too irritable to enjoy their customary card games; they became too listless and lethargic to exercise; their waking thoughts—and even their dreams—converged on food. Obviously, weight loss had serious repercussions on these otherwise healthy volunteers.

One interpretation of the negative impact of this self-imposed "diet" is that the subjects were "psychologically frustrated." They were given food but could never get quite enough. This situation may be a form of mental torture, with the various mental and behavioral "pathologies" emerging as a response to this distress. The fact that, as time and weight loss progressed, it required even greater feats of abstinence to achieve minor incremental weight loss—and that for some people, weight loss resisted all their exertions—would make the situation all the more frustrating. True enough. But consider a different question: Why did weight loss slow down and in some cases stop altogether? Was this sabotage of the research objective purely psychological, or was there something more involved? Subjects claimed to be trying; and, indeed, their caloric restriction did not let up any. Yet weight loss slowed and in some cases stopped before the goal was achieved. Might there be something nonpsychological at work to inhibit weight loss? Something physiological? Does the body, perhaps, actively resist attempts to alter weight too dramatically?

Prisons are not noted for their haute cuisine. Between the forced exercise and the at best tolerable food, inmates generally need to let out their frustrations more often than the seams on their clothing. A group of prisoners in Vermont in the 1960s, however, found themselves in an extraordinary situation—they volunteered for a study on obesity and found themselves being encouraged to get fat, and not just with verbal exhortations. They were provided with tasty food—much better than standard prison chow—and plenty of it. Their task was to *increase* their weight by about a quarter, so they were given extra food, milkshakes, cakes, and other high calorie treats. In all, they consumed two or three times their normal caloric intake each day. Some of the men had no trouble gaining weight, and gradually reached their overweight goal. Most of them, however, found it difficult to reach the target weight, and some were simply unable to do so. For some prisoners, adding pounds was not as easy as it had originally sounded. Worse yet, as the prisoners' weight increased, their energy, activity, and initiative all declined. In another study, four college students were paid to gain as much as they could. Despite systematic overeating of rich, good-tasting food, they were able to increase their weight only by about 10 percent in 3–5 months. And, finally, in France there is an organization called the Hundred Kilo Club. Membership is restricted to those weighing at least 100 kilograms, or 220 pounds. It seems there are a number of

200-pound Frenchmen and Frenchwomen who have been striving in vain for some time to reach the 100-kilo level in order to join the club—and they just can't do it.

One can only wonder about what might be inhibiting weight gain in these various situations, each characterized by good food, lots of motivation, and no evident reason not to succeed. One could perhaps devise a "mental" explanation for the sabotage of the weight gain attempt—for example, an "unconscious fear of fatness." As with the Minnesota weight losers, however, these ambitious weight gainers found that a diet that was initially adequate to the task—that did, in fact, cause weight to change in the desired direction—gradually lost its efficacy. One is again tempted to speculate about possible physiological mechanisms designed to inhibit excessive weight change—in either direction.

How much do you weigh? How much should you weigh? How much would you weigh if you could weigh whatever you wanted? For some people, the answer to all three questions is the same. For most of us, though, there is a gap between what we actually weigh and what we would like to weigh. In fact, for some of us there's even a gap between what we think we should weigh and what we'd like to weigh. After all, it wouldn't hurt to be a little "underweight," would it? A few pounds below ideal weight might be the buffer we need to protect us from the effects of the occasional splurge.

Isn't it strange that there is so often a gap between where we are in terms of weight and where we'd like to be? Considering that we have control over our weight level, why are so many of us dissatisfied with it? Of all the dissatisfactions with our appearance that we can identify, dissatisfaction with weight is probably the most universal—certainly the most pervasive in our culture. Why should this be so? It is our thesis that weight is an especially ambiguous element of appearance, in terms of whether or not we can control it; and it is this ambiguity— basically, our belief that we can and should control it, combined with our frequently evident lack of control over it—that makes weight such a psychologically "loaded" and frustrating aspect of appearance.

There are, of course, many elements of appearance that are not really amenable to significant change; and one would think that being "stuck with" an unsatisfactory attribute (such as big feet, or a big nose) might be particularly galling. We are all expert, however, in adjusting to the inevitable; for the most part, we don't even think about our big feet and/or noses, just as we don't especially bemoan our inability to flap our arms and fly, even though the otherwise less sophisticated birds can do so. We learn to face facts. It is only those conditions for which there is a realistic hope of improvement that preoccupy us. (We don't mean to slight the concerns that some people do have over certain unalterable aspects of appearance. The short man may show continuing concern about his "unfair" condition. But such continuing concern is not the typical response to shortness, whereas, when it comes to weight, a majority of people seem to be actively, vocally dissatisfied.)

The fact that weight seems potentially changeable or improvable, then, accounts in part for the widespread dissatisfaction. But, obviously, the possibility of improving something shouldn't result in *continuing* dissatisfaction. One can always go ahead and make the improvements, removing the bothersome gap between one's actual condition and one's desired condition. Many elements of our appearance, in fact, are remarkably susceptible to change; the beauty shop—not to mention the plastic surgeon—provides ample evidence of that. But the majority of people *don't* seek plastic surgery.

The problem with weight, then, is not so much whether or not it can be changed as that our notions of *how much* or *how easily* it can be changed tend to exceed the true facts of the matter. Weight can indeed be changed, which is why we concern ourselves with it and try to effect those changes; however, it is not as changeable as most of us would like to believe. Thus, our reach tends to exceed our grasp where weight loss is concerned. Frustration and dissatisfaction are the understandable consequences.

How has this situation come about? Why do we underestimate the difficulty of losing weight? For the most part, this underestimation is due to a widespread axiom in our culture—namely, that weight is one of those elements of appearance that is more or less arbitrary and therefore subject to almost unlimited change.

An analogy with a bank account may be instructive. We can withdraw money from our account, right down to the point where the account is empty. Likewise, we can easily add whatever amount we have on hand. We view our weight, then, as analogous to our bank account balance: it can move up and down freely, depending only on the amounts we choose to withdraw or deposit.

Yet, obviously, losing weight is a lot harder than withdrawing money; we all know that from experience. But why? Where does the analogy break down? What is the difference between the bank account and our weight "account" (calculated, naturally, in pounds)?

We shall argue that the difference stems from two characteristics of weight, characteristics of which the public has a vague sense but not a proper appreciation (for reasons we'll discuss later). These characteristics are the following:

1. There are enduring individual differences in what we may call "natural weight."

2. These "natural weights" are biologically (and biobehaviorally) defended.

Let us examine these propositions in some detail, beginning with the term "natural weight." What we mean by this term is that for each individual there is a particular weight that is most natural or comfortable. (The term "natural weight" is roughly equivalent to the concept of "set point" as used in research on regulation. Set point, however, tends to be used with reference to a particular weight, whereas we use natural weight to convey the notion of a broader range of regulated weight.) We shall discuss later how this particular range is determined; for now, suffice it to say that it exists, and that it provides a "biological goal" toward which our bodies strive, with more or less vigor. Departures from one's natural weight are not impossible; in fact, they are frequent. Each departure, however, activates a "biobehavioral defense system," as reflected in our second proposition above. It may well be the case that small departures incur little or no resistance (defense), but large departures virtually always stimulate a spirited (and dispiriting) defense. These defenses entail a full range of biological and behavioral adjustments—changes in our metabolism, our perceptions of food, our emotions, and, of course, our eating. (The changes in eating, which is ultimately a voluntary behavior, are not automatic; however, if you make a horse thirsty enough, then leading him to water will virtually *compel* him to drink.) These defenses are designed specifically to prevent undue departures from one's natural weight. (Actually, there is some argument as to whether it is weight per se that is defended, or fat. This distinction, although of interest to scientists, does not make much difference for our present purposes, since weight and fat levels rise and fall pretty much in tandem. Some weight change, as is well known, reflects fluctuations in our bodily storage of water. Probably a good part of the daily weight fluctuations we all experience involves some water gain or loss, depending on our particular diet and physical activity patterns. Nevertheless, most substantial changes—that is, changes of more than 5 pounds—in body weight over more than a day or two involve changes in stored fat levels. In what follows, we shall continue to speak as if it is weight that is being defended; we must recognize, however, that it may well be fat that is the true object of physiological defense.)

To resume our bank account analogy, it is as if someone decided that our bank account should contain $1,000. (Less than $1,000 doesn't provide a sufficient margin of security; and more than $1,000 is unnecessary and wasteful, since the money could be more profitably invested elsewhere.) Deposits or withdrawals are permitted, as long as the balance stays in the range of $1,000 plus or minus $50. (It goes without saying that these dollar figures are arbitrary and selected only for illustrative purposes. A permissible range of plus or minus 5 percent around the defended level, however, seems to be fairly realistic when it comes to weight—though, as we'll see, some people's accounts have a wider permissible range than do others'.) If one attempts to make a withdrawal that would leave less than $950 in the account, the bank's computer objects. It does not absolutely prohibit further withdrawals, but it makes them difficult. For instance, it may be programmed so that for every further dollar you try to withdraw, it releases only fifty cents. As withdrawals continue, it may gradually reduce the fraction released until eventually it stops releasing money altogether. As dieters know, the first few pounds are usually the easiest to lose; further weight loss becomes progressively more difficult.

Other strategies used by the bank's computer in defending the $1,000 balance against inordinate withdrawals might include making you aware, perhaps through some sort of subliminal manipulation, of irresistible cravings to deposit money. It may arrange things so that making deposits is especially satisfying; it may even sweeten things by arranging to augment deposits, so that, if your balance is too low, for each dollar you deposit the bank will add a contribution of its own. (Imagine a situation where all deposits are subject to some "wastage" in the form of a service charge imposed by the bank. If your balance falls too low, however, the bank can reduce or even eliminate this charge, in effect increasing the value of your deposits, until your balance is back in the optimal range.)

If laboratory rats are starved down significantly below their "natural weight"—the weight that they would ordinarily maintain on standard lab chow (with standard, minimal exercise)—they will, not surprisingly, consume more food when it's available, to bring their weight back up to what it "should" be. What is surprising is that the starved-down rat also *gains* weight on a *restricted* diet. In short, being starved down below natural weight affects the rat's metabolism in such a way that the calories that *are* ingested go further, metabolically. It's as if the animal extracts more of the *potential* energy contained in those calories—and calories, after all, are measured in terms of their potential energy value if they are burned completely, which is not necessarily the case in the average organism. A weight reduction below the natural range, then, may shift metabolism in an anabolic ("fattening") direction, by causing ingested calories to be used more efficiently. The result is what has often been referred to as a thrifty metabolism (making the most of what one eats). Thus, the analogy of a wasteful service charge, which can be revoked if the bank's plan is to augment deposits, is not so far off the mark.

Another way of decreasing normal wastage is to alter heat expenditure. Part of the energy that we expend is dissipated in a process known as nonshivering thermogenesis (heat production), which is apparently determined by the activity of brown fat deposits in the body. Animals with a greater amount of active brown fat—or whose brown fat is more active—literally burn off more calories in what amounts to wastage. When animals are starved down, however, the heat-generating activity of their brown fat is reduced, in what may be regarded as a physiological program of energy conservation. Again, the physiology of the animal below his natural weight range conspires to eliminate energy wastage, in an apparent attempt to restore weight to its natural (physiologically optimal) level. Yet again, the notion of a service charge, ordinarily wasteful but subject to revocation under conditions where the system cannot afford any more waste, seems useful.

This analogy, of course, has its deficiencies; one obvious example is that the weight defense/regulation system operates internally and doesn't require an outside monitor and regulator (such as a computer). Of course, we do use the bathroom scale, which is obviously an outside monitor. Such a device permits one to judge the extent to which one's weight departs from the intended weight; as a consequence, one may attempt to take corrective action. In this case, however, the intended weight —the weight toward which the individual consciously strives —is not necessarily the same weight that is defended *biologically*. (Indeed, it is the very fact that we defend one weight with our bodies and another weight with our heads that produces the problems that this book addresses.)

The Defense of Natural Weight

Most individuals regard the term "weight problem" as synonymous with "overweight." In other words, most people trying to change their weight are trying to lose. The notion of body weight defense, however, operates in both directions. Thus, one may have little trouble making deposits up to $1,050; indeed, if you start from a point below your optimal balance of $1,000, the bank may augment your deposits, as we've seen. Above $1,050, however, deposits (i.e., further departures from the defended value) become increasingly difficult. Attempts to deposit a dollar produce actual deposits of only a fraction of that amount owing to sharply increased service charges; and, as the balance slowly increases, the fraction may decline to the point where further increases in the balance are virtually impossible. At the same time, the would-be depositor may be overwhelmed by a desire to make a withdrawal—and may find that the bank withdraws more from the account than was intended. The same processes that are engaged to conserve energy when weight drops too low can be reversed when weight rises too high. Thus, more of the calories that are ingested can be metabolically unused or wasted, and more, rather than less, heat wastage can be achieved through brown fat nonshivering thermogenesis. In short, the system is bidirectional, as it must be if it is to defend a particular weight range from excessive deviations in either direction.

But isn't it the case that our weight jumps around? Everyone knows that if we are exposed to especially good food, our weight will rise ("tracking" our intake); with bad food, the opposite occurs. Rats and humans, it is true, show weight variation in response to changes in the palatability of their diets. However, the important point is that these changes are not unregulated. We can move only so far. Thus, although good (or bad) food presents a challenge to our defenses and may shift our weight to the limit those defenses allow, such shifts shouldn't be seen as reflecting the absence of defenses.

Although the very notion of defense implies that one's natural weight is defended from departures in either direction (i.e., from significant weight gain *and* loss), it is not necessarily the case that the defense is perfectly symmetrical. That is, it is possible for a particular weight range to be defended, but for the defense to be especially vigorous against, say, weight loss. Significant upward departures may instigate defensive reactions, but less quickly and/or less powerfully. In other words, nature may prefer that one maintain an optimal (natural) weight, but show less concern about one type of failure (weight gain) than another (weight loss), presumably because the latter poses a more immediate and/or serious threat to survival.

Our discussion of how weight *can* change, despite the operation of built-in defenses, returns us to our original concern about the basis for society's frustration over weight. Weight regulation, in the last analysis, is ambiguous with respect to the potential for change: it all depends on whether we're struck by people's evident capacity to achieve desired change or by their inability to do so. If we develop a belief in the possibility of unlimited change, we are bound to be disappointed. If we develop a belief in the impossibility of change, the evidence of our senses will contradict that belief.

We see all around us people undergoing weight changes— deliberate or otherwise. In fact, some people show tremendous variability in their weights. On the other hand, some overweight people change little, but perhaps that's because they don't try hard enough. The basic problem—the problem underlying our collective frustration—is our incoherent collective interpretation of the weight changes (and nonchanges) we observe.

The Defense of Natural Weight

Consider two individuals, A and B, who are of the same sex, same height, and same weight. Both consider themselves a little overweight, and both decide to lose 15 pounds. Although they both adopt the same restricted diet and exercise regimen, A loses weight more easily and rapidly than B. What are we to conclude from this? One possibility is that A and/or B are deviating from the program, so that A ends up eating less and/or exercising more than B. As it's usually very difficult to obtain accurate observations of caloric intake or expenditure, such a possibility may be quite plausible. After all, there are good reasons (eagerness, competitiveness) for A to speed things up, and good reasons, or at least plausible reasons (laziness, weakness of the flesh) for B to slow things down. As often as not people tend to make these psychological or behavioral interpretations of individual differences in outcome. Such interpretations ultimately boil down to the assertion that A and B are losing weight at different rates because, quite simply, they are achieving different caloric input–output ratios. Somewhere along the line, A is sneaking ahead; or, more likely, B, through some sort of personal weakness, is falling behind the planned rate of loss. These inferences are based on the time-honored notion that a calorie is a calorie, and that if A is losing more than B, then it's because A is consuming fewer and/or expending more net calories.

We feel that this "calorie is a calorie" principle has its limits. We accept it insofar as it means that a calorie of lettuce equals a calorie of fudge. However, as we have indicated, it does not seem to be true that a calorie (of fudge *or* lettuce) will necessarily have the same effect on A as on B (or C or D . . .). Thus, to return to our bank account analogy, we do not accept this principle insofar as it implies that a deposit of a dollar in A's account has the same effect as a deposit of a dollar in B's account. We have seen that one of the mechanisms available to counteract departures from one's optimal level is adjustment of the effect of attempted deposits, and that, whereas for someone above the optimal level the deposit will be reduced by the defense system, for someone below the optimal level the deposit will be augmented. Put back into caloric terms, we do not mean to imply that fractional quantities of what we eat mysteriously come and go; rather, we mean to imply that by the time a calorie of fudge passes through A's metabolic system, there may be more or less of it left for storage as fat (relative to what its fate may be in B's metabolic system). Thus, the fact that A loses weight more quickly than does B may well reflect a true biological difference between them—A's system is less anabolic (fat storage prone) than is B's.

But why should that be? After all, A and B both started at the same weight, and they are of the same height and sex. Why should A be blessed with a less anabolic system and B cursed with a more anabolic system? If both start with $1,000 in their accounts, they should have equal ease/difficulty in withdrawing, say, $100. Must we assume, confusingly, that A's balance is less well defended than B's? The answer is yes and no.

It is reasonable to assume that the particular balance of $1,000 elicits a weaker defensive reaction in A than in B; losing, say, $75 is clearly easier for A. But we must be careful to remember that the fact that A and B share a common gender, height, and (initial) weight does not imply that their *defended weights* (i.e., natural weights) are equivalent. If A and B both start at 140 pounds, and set out to lose 15 pounds, the fact that A has an easier time of it may mean, quite simply, that A's natural weight is 120 pounds, whereas B's is 140. If that were the case, we'd expect A to have a much easier time: for

A, losing weight is congruent with weight defense; for B, it is incongruent.

Even if A's natural weight were 130 pounds, it would still prove easier for A to lose the 15 desired pounds: the first 10 pounds would not elicit any defensive opposition at all, metabolically; and the next 5 pounds probably wouldn't elicit *much* opposition. For B, though, 15 pounds below natural weight is a lot. Five pounds mightn't provoke much defense. But those next 10 pounds are likely to be very difficult.

Finally, let's imagine that A's natural weight is 140. If so, A should have trouble. But, B's natural weight might be 150, in which case B's troubles would make A's pale by comparison. By now the point should be obvious. If A and B start from the same *actual* weight, but have different *natural* weights (A's being lower), then A will have relatively less trouble losing than will B. If A's starting weight is *above* A's natural weight—which is possible, though perhaps not likely—then A's defense system will actually encourage weight loss, down to the level of natural weight. In our society, many dieters start off from a position *at* or *below* their natural weight. Even if that's the case for A, though, A's weight loss attempt, while not necessarily pleasant, will be easier than B's if B's natural weight is higher than A's. In short, if two people, starting from the same weight level, set out to lose weight, the person with the lower natural weight will have the advantage—regardless of whether he or she starts from above, below, or right at his or her natural weight level. The same principle applies, in reverse, to attempts at weight gain. Consider girls with anorexia nervosa, a self-starvation syndrome we discuss in a later chapter. Often, by the time the patient gets hospital treatment, her weight has dropped so low that death from starvation is a real possibility.

The immediate need is for weight gain, so patients are induced or even forced to eat, or "refeed." It has often been observed that patients at roughly the same weight—say, 70 pounds—require dramatically different numbers of calories to achieve a weight of, say, 90 pounds. One predictor of weight gain per calorie is pre-anorexic weight—the higher the original weight, the easier, calorically, it is to gain. Another way of looking at this is that the 70-pounder who used to weigh 130 is in some respects more "underweight"—further below natural weight—than is the 70-pounder who used to weigh 110. It stands to reason that the ex-130-pounder's body would exhibit a stronger anabolic adjustment than would the ex-110-pounder's. This difference, then, boils down to the issue of natural weight location, and how far one is from it.

Furthermore, as we will discuss in more detail a bit later, people differ not only in natural weight levels, but also in how broad a range their natural weights cover, and in how rigidly or loosely their natural weights are defended by their bodies. In other words, some people have broad ranges of weight which their bodies will tolerate or find comfortable—say, a 20 pound spread—while others have a narrower band of acceptable weights—say, a 3–5 pound spread. And some bodies fight vigorously to stay within their natural weight boundaries, whereas other bodies are more flexible about weight deviations, tolerating larger departures from their optimal natural weight levels.

So far, we've been rather vague about exactly what the defenses are that make weight loss so much more difficult for B than for A. We've suggested that one level of defense is metabolic; that is, the physiological processes involved in converting our food intake to energy, and the heat/energy mechanics involved in caloric expenditure, may differ according to whether one is above, below, or at one's natural weight. (And, if A and B are *both* below but B more so than A, then the metabolic defense will be more severe for B; defensive activity is not an all-or-none phenomenon, but more a matter of degree—and direction.)

Studies on laboratory rats have demonstrated, as we've seen, that food deprivation induces caloric thrift. Likewise, severe weight gain is often accompanied by the opposite metabolic tendency, catabolism, wherein energy is spent more freely than usual. In either case, a calorie is not a calorie—at least when we abandon the perspective of thinking about calories in terms of energy potential (i.e., the calorie counter approach) and adopt a more realistic view of calories as *actually realized* energy. It is important that we attend to the issue of what we *do* to the calories contained in food, rather than just focusing on those calories in the abstract.

Metabolism, of course, is not the sort of thing over which we have much personal control. (It is true that we can take drugs to influence our metabolic rate and by "burning off" more calories, promote weight loss. However, no such drug has proven to be both safe and effective.) It may well be the very fact that metabolic adjustments are *not* subject to deliberate control that makes them nature's choice for the ultimate defense. The best defense is one we cannot readily interfere with. (Perhaps these considerations bear on the general issue of drug or hormonal interventions in weight control and why they are ultimately so ineffective. Nature uses metabolic rate to defend natural weight. If we seek to fool that defense pharmacologically, we may succeed for a while—but nature will not idly tolerate the negation of one of its major defense systems. It will either bolster the defense, rendering the drug relatively ineffective over time—which is what usually happens—or fall back on another defensive strategy such as illness tied to drug use, necessitating the discontinuance of the drug.)

Other defenses are more accessible to our intervention. For instance, if an anabolic tendency toward fat storage is one prime defense mechanism, another might involve promptings to increase net caloric balance (which would lessen the need for anabolism). Increasing the number of calories available for fat storage might involve a defense whereby active exercising was discouraged. If weight loss were to produce fatigue or lethargy, then it's likely that fewer calories would be expended in voluntary exercise; if intake were held constant, the net effect would be a caloric increase. In humans, certainly, one of the most common effects of severe food deprivation is equally severe lethargy, which clearly serves to conserve what little energy is available.

Reducing caloric expenditure, of course, is not the only means available for increasing the net balance of calories in the system. Perhaps the easiest way to add calories is to eat rich foods; and, while nature can't force us to eat, she can make life pretty miserable (and eating correspondingly pleasant) for the underweight individual. Hunger is generally an aversive sensation, as it should be since it's designed to prompt us to eat. Those who have undergone serious weight loss report that they experience hunger more often and/or more intensely. Likewise, the pleasure of eating may change, so that the taste of food improves for the person attempting un-natural weight loss. More food can be eaten, and it tastes better longer.

Normally, although we enjoy sweet tastes, a lot of sweetness becomes aversive when it's experienced over a short time span, with no relief. Physiologists use the term "alliesthesia" to denote changes in the pleasantness of sensations; negative alliesthesia refers to the decline in our preference for sweets as we consume more of them (over a short period of time). In the laboratory, the process is often telescoped by having the experimental subject consume a large "load" of glucose solution; the preference for sweets (as represented by a liking for different concentrations of sugar water) drops dramatically after the glucose load. Some experimental subjects, however, fail to show the normal reaction to the glucose load. Despite massive exposure to sweet taste, their preference for it remains high. Close examination of these subjects indicates that in most cases they are people whom we have reason to believe are below their natural weight. Similarly, when a group of researchers lost 10 percent of their own body weights over a period of weeks, their negative alliesthesia disappeared as they lost the weight. With subsequent weight gain, the reaction returned. This dynamic phenomenon is a splendid example of how nature defends against unwanted weight changes. When people lose weight, their sweet preference in effect increases. They're more likely to want that sweet dessert—and more likely to want a second helping after the first. This abnormal reaction lasts only as long as weight remains suppressed. Recovery of one's natural weight eliminates the need for this perceptual defense mechanism. (It should be noted, however, that this defensive sweet tooth may be more easy to acquire than to lose. There is some evidence that it may persist even after weight recovery, or after weight stabilization in subjects who are observed only during weight gain. It may well prove to be the case that anabolic defenses are easier to turn on than to turn off, as we suggested earlier when discussing the probable asymmetry in defense favoring weight gain. These issues are far from settled, but some researchers are coming to believe that ex-dieters tend to gain to a weight even higher than their starting point, owing to the persistent aftereffects of metabolic and other defenses geared to counteract the effects of the diet.)

Eating and lethargy as defense mechanisms are effective, in their way; sometimes they are overly effective, as we've seen, but they are also fallible. With sufficient dedication, one can train oneself to ignore hunger (or at least not respond to it by overeating), to resist even the most tasty food, to jog despite exhaustion. The success of these mechanisms thus depends on whether their promptings—the pleasures and pains they confer for doing or not doing something in the interest of restoring natural weight—can be overcome by personal dedication. Pain and pleasure are powerful determinants of behavior, as we know. But, except in the most extreme cases, they are not absolutely compelling. People can act *despite* pleasure or pain if their "will" is strong enough. For the weak-willed dieter, these forces may be enough to prevent excessive deviation from natural weight. For the strong-willed dieter, though, defenses dependent on overt behavior may not suffice. If the dieter refuses to eat enough or to exercise less rigorously, nature may have to fall back on the more reliable, less disruptible defenses like metabolic adjustment.

The fact that there are so many different defenses available for the protection of natural weight may be discouraging to the individual trying to "escape" his or her natural weight. If we remain objective, though, we should be struck by the fact that natural weight *is* so well defended. It is plausible to interpret this multiplicity of defenses as strong evidence for the biological importance of natural weight; nature protects that which is most valuable. But what *is* the biological value of natural weight?

The answer to this question isn't all that clear. Scientists tend to work backwards, inferring importance from defense. That is, if something is so well protected, it must be valuable. This reasoning may not appear particularly logical, but it accords, at least, with our essentially functional view of nature. People may act irrationally, valuing what is valueless, but nature, owing to the pressures of natural selection, values what is valuable. And since natural weight is evidently valued (i.e., defended) so intensely, it must serve a useful evolutionary purpose.

The evolutionary purposes of an attribute are difficult to detect except in the particular habitat or ecological niche for which that attribute was designed. Thus it is important to keep reminding ourselves that we, on this continent, are a heterogeneous society in terms of our geographic and racial backgrounds. While we inhabit (more or less) the same environment now, we may be genetically programmed for vastly different environments. Climate, the availability and reliability of food sources, and various other constraints on our internal energy supply, all contributed to our forefathers' evolving physiques—and these physiques are passed on to us, whether we want them or not, and whether they suit our "lifestyle" or not. Intermarriage and breeding across genetic pools complicate matters, producing gradations of diversity. The defense of natural weight, then, may be interpreted as a natural protection for the organism, an adaptation to an ecological niche. Individual differences in the weight that is defended may correspond to our different "niches of origin."

Even within a particular niche, though, we encounter some diversity of defended weights in different individuals. Diversity is usually seen as evolutionarily advantageous—to the group, if not to the individual—since it virtually guarantees that *some* members of the larger group will be suitably adapted to whatever environmental disturbances they may face. Thus, the defense of diverse natural weights provides protection to the group within a particular niche; and any society whose members' ancestors inhabited widely varying niches will show all the more diversity in defended natural weights.

In any case, we must recognize that different natural weights are represented (and defended) in the population. Furthermore, as has been mentioned, there also appears to be individual variation in the intensity of natural weight defenses (as well as in their symmetry and perhaps other parameters). Thus, even if two people defend the same natural weight, and start from the same point—say, right at the natural weight optimal level—one might find it easier to lose than does the other. The difference between them is not in defended natural weight, but in the vigor of the defense—as if nature objects to, and takes action against, deviations from optimal weight to a greater extent in some people than in others. Another way of looking at this difference is that some people's defenses are activated when a small deviation occurs, whereas others' remain inactive until a larger deviation takes place. In this view, the difference isn't a matter of intensity of defense but *at what point* the defense begins. At present, the two views are almost impossible to disentangle scientifically; and it is certainly possible that people differ with respect to *both* intensity and the onset point (or range) of defense (as well as with respect to natural weight itself). Regardless of these qualifications, though, it is *not* a matter of biological indifference what an individual weighs. And the important criterion for what constitutes an appropriate weight is not what "everyone else" weighs, but what one's own internal (natural weight) standards dictate. These dictates aren't all powerful, as we've seen—but they're not impotent either. If one undertakes to achieve a weight significantly different from the one intended and defended physiologically, one will almost certainly incur discomfort; and, even if one is willing to put up with discomfort, one may still fail.

An additional twist to the problem involves the possibility, as we've seen, that repeated serious attempts to change one's weight from its natural level may produce backlash effects. Thus, the individual who tries to lose 15 pounds may, when the effort to keep that weight off is relaxed, bounce back up to a level even higher than the starting point. It's as if, in order to protect a weight of, say, 140 pounds from repeated attempts to diet, nature builds in an extra cushion, maintaining weight above the original natural weight of 140 pounds. There is a small amount of evidence for this "overshooting." For example, the conscientious objectors described earlier regained, at least initially, to 105 percent of their original weight. Moreover, a higher percentage of the regained weight was fat tissue as compared to pre-weight-loss body composition. Little is understood at present about these "anticipatory" defensive adjustments; however, it appears to be the case that the body has a memory, and keeps track of whether it houses the sort of person who will require extra precautionary measures to keep in check. We believe that through such mechanisms repeated dieting has actually *raised* the weight of many of its practitioners.

We have presented the case for the existence of a natural, defended weight as if, through genetic transmission, one is at birth bequeathed a magic number which remains in force throughout one's life. One can alter one's actual weight up or down, and various defenses can work to compensate (or overcompensate) for these shifts; however, the natural weight around which these shifts occur, and which limits the extent of these shifts, remains constant once adulthood is reached—

and was presumably already programmed, like one's eventual height, earlier in life.

We should hasten to add, however, that many aspects of natural weight remain uncertain or unknown. For instance, we cannot measure natural weight directly, but rather must *infer* it from (a) what happens when one's weight is allowed to "float" freely, and/or (b) the difficulties that one encounters in trying to rise above or fall below a particular weight. In short, we infer natural weight from the effects of the defenses that maintain it; and we locate natural weight at the point where the defenses subside.

Just as we can't really measure natural weight directly, so we are uncertain about the physiological processes that underly it. Even granting that individual differences in natural weight are of genetic origin, we must confess to considerable ignorance about what structures or processes "contain the information" as to what one's natural weight is. It was thought—and still is, by some—that natural weight was "determined" by the number of fat cells we developed, which in turn reflected both genetic and nutritional influences. There is certainly a strong positive correlation between the number of fat cells (adipocytes) one has and the weight one seems to defend. Differences in fat cell number between people, then, may correspond to differences in their natural weights. Differences in fat cell size, on the other hand, presumably reflect variations in actual fat storage rather than in natural weight. Dieting should reduce average cell size without affecting cell number, since it affects actual weight, not natural weight.

The foregoing argument, unfortunately, is rather speculative. As it happens, problems with the identification and measurement of fat cells have arisen. Furthermore, it appears to be the case that changing the number of fat cells does not necessarily produce a corresponding change in defended weight level. Obese mice, for instance, despite lipectomy—the surgical removal of fat tissue—nevertheless managed to return eventually to their preoperative weight. This suggests that the "code" for natural weight doesn't lie in the fat cells themselves. Thus, there is currently less enthusiasm for the view that the number of fat cells is the fundamental basis of natural weight.

Another candidate for the "carrier" of natural weight is the brown fat involved in nonshivering thermogenesis. There appear to be wide individual differences in the activity of brown fat pads; individuals with especially active brown fat will tend to be leaner, all things being equal, since they tend to burn off more food energy. Likewise, it has been suggested that some forms of obesity may result from "defects" in the functioning of brown fat, with excess energy accumulating as a consequence of inactive (or insufficient) brown fat. The researchers involved have been suitably cautious in their analysis of the role of brown fat, but like fat cells a decade ago, brown fat has great potential for public mystification. The fact that a particular tissue contributes to the regulation of weight seems to suggest —at least to a desperate minority—that here, finally, is the answer. One can imagine an exploitive entrepreneur marketing a diet or mechanical advice designed to "activate" one's "lazy" brown fat—and thus painlessly promote weight loss while the patient eats all he or she wants! If one could increase the activity of brown fat without changing anything else this weight loss fantasy might not be so implausible. However, the problem is not just to activate the brown fat; one must also ensure that no compensatory reactions occur to balance out the change in brown fat activity. We must remember that these metabolic activities evidently occur *in the service of* natural weight. If one agent (e.g., brown fat) isn't doing its defensive job, it may be replaced—or overwhelmed—by another agent. Opening the window on a winter's day, remember, does not lower the setting on the thermostat; it just makes the furnace work harder. Brown fat may eventually prove to be manipulable without compensatory defensive consequences; however, we have seen enough "breakthroughs"—attempts to circumvent the basis for weight regulation at a level too high for the individual's personal satisfaction—to be skeptical. Meaningful permanent changes in the body's level of natural weight will require a clearer understanding of the *determinants* of natural weight than we have at present.

Looking at the issue from a more optimistic perspective, we may note that our ignorance about the biological basis and mechanisms of natural weight permits us to indulge the possibility that the "setting" for natural weight might change (or be changed). Some have argued that changes do occur "spontaneously"—which is to say, for reasons that we don't understand. Others have argued that a major hormonal upheaval (such as occurs during adolescence or pregnancy) may permanently alter one's natural weight.

Obviously, if we had any reliable information about the determinants of (changes in) natural weight, the prospects for dieters might be improved. If we could "change the setting" for natural weight, then weight loss might be congruent rather than incongruent with our physiological requirements, and it wouldn't elicit aversive defensive reactions. Perhaps, as research progresses, we will eventually be able to imagine such biological interventions—even including genetic manipulations. For now, though, and for the foreseeable future, we must resign ourselves to the fact that we have no reliable way to change the natural weight that an individual is blessed or cursed with. If one is dissatisfied with one's weight, one can

The Defense of Natural Weight

only try the time-honored techniques of weight change—with all the defensive reactions and discomforts that they typically involve. If there is any consolation to be derived from our present state of knowledge, it's that comparisons with other people probably don't make any biological sense. They certainly shouldn't be used as a basis for evaluating one's character. If others have more or less trouble altering weight than we do, they are probably the beneficiaries or victims of a different —more or less fortunate—natural weight. Character enters into it, of course, since the weak-willed person can't hope to make headway in the fight against biological defenses—but all the will in the world won't help if there isn't a biological way.

CHAPTER 3

Overweight, Overeating, and Health

T HE DEFENSE of natural weight poses problems for dieters intent on losing pounds which their bodies struggle to retain. By the same token, dieting poses problems for the defense of natural weight. It seems evident that if one's natural weight and one's ideal (target) weight are seriously discrepant, then one or the other must be sacrificed. It is this sacrifice that makes dieting such a difficult and frustrating undertaking.

That there is a need for sacrifice at all, of course, reflects the fact that there is so often an apparent gap between natural and ideal weights. In the previous chapter we discussed natural weight and its defense. In the next few chapters we shall focus on ideals.

We are all familiar with charts of ideal weights, adjusted for sex, height, and occasionally general stature. The charts themselves, however, rarely describe how these ideals are arrived at, nor what they are ideal for. What does it mean to be at an "ideal" weight? Obviously, it doesn't mean being at one's natural weight; if it did, then most of us would be perfectly content with our weight. What, then, are these "unnatural" ideals?

Basically, the ideal weight is defined in two ways: medical and cultural. (The fact that there are two ideals means that there is room for conflict even at the ideal level.) In this chapter, we shall examine the medical ideals that provide the motive for so much desperate dieting. Not everyone who diets does so primarily in order to become healthier, as we shall see; but improved health is usually regarded as at least a welcome side effect of weight loss. And, for many fat, middle-aged men, the alleged health benefits of dieting *are* paramount. Undeniably, then, the attempt to achieve good health—or at least to avoid disease and quite possibly premature death—is often a primary and compelling goal of dieting. As we have heard countless times, obesity is America's number one health problem. (So are smoking, drinking, venereal disease, and mental illness—but why quibble?)

The first question we must ask is, why would nature, after going to all the trouble of arranging for the intricate and tenacious defense of natural weight, allow a situation in which maintaining your natural weight could perhaps prove fatal? We have argued that some people are naturally fatter than are others. Are these people the victims of some sort of biological accident, with a natural weight so high as to represent a risk to life itself? That doesn't make much biological sense. Evolutionary theorists, however, have managed (as usual) to come up with an explanation for this apparent biological anomaly. The argument is as follows: In historical epochs when the food supply was severely limited or unreliable, a large amount of body fat was an advantage in bridging the often lengthy famines between feasts. Likewise, the tendency to put on more weight during and after those feasts—in modern metabolic terms, anabolism—was also a decided advantage. It might thus plausibly happen that natural selection would favor those with a high natural weight. (These are the same people who would become particularly anabolic during famines.) The favoritism shown by natural selection toward fat, however, is premised on a situation of ecological scarcity; under such conditions, fatness promotes life, since starvation is a real threat, and even a mere subsistence diet may not provide individuals with enough strength to withstand disease or other predations. Even in such circumstances, a large accumulation of fat might well prove to be medically dangerous, as is alleged to be the case in our society. But conditions of scarcity, while favoring fat, rarely allowed for its excessive accumulation; famine usually prevailed over feast. And most of those who lived long enough to die from the sorts of disorders usually associated with overweight considered themselves lucky. On balance, the survival advantages of fat outweighed its disadvantages.

In contrast, the argument continues, starvation is not a threat to most members of today's industrial societies. Indeed, the abundance that nature programmed us to take advantage of during its previously rare appearances is now chronic. Our ecological niche has changed much more rapidly than our genetic adaptation to it. We are built for scarcity, yet we live in plenty. Obesity is the unfortunate result. And, because the health hazards of obesity are often delayed until well into or beyond the childbearing years, "obese genes" are not selected out of the gene pool. The threat of obesity, then, is not lifelong, but tends to appear initially in one's forties or fifties. By the standards of civilizations past, that's not too bad; in present-day industrial societies, though, most of us feel entitled to reach our seventies or eighties.

The foregoing analysis suggests that obesity emerges as a problem only in societies of abundance (and reasonably long life expectancy). Still, this analysis does not provide any real explanation of *why* being fat ought to be a problem at all, medically. Fat people can't move as fast as their slimmer counterparts, perhaps—but, then again, our society probably demands less physical speed and agility than did any of its predecessors. Fat people may have more trouble finding a mate (for "esthetic" reasons), but that's not a medical problem. When doctors dispense the advice, ". . . and you could stand to lose a few pounds," what exactly is their concern? And, when doctors inform patients that overweight is literally killing them, what facts underlie this assertion?

THE DANGERS OF OVERWEIGHT

The charted ideal weights for sex and height are for the most part based on actuarial analyses of mortality and morbidity— which is to say, they represent the weights at which individuals, aggregated across large samples, are least likely to encounter death or the disabling diseases against which they are insured. As is now well known, these figures are based on an unrepresentative sample of the general population (namely, those who sought life insurance and were deemed eligible). Thus, such ideal figures might change somewhat if the entire population were considered. More problematic, though, is the fact that these ideal values are not based on any sort of scientific, causal analysis; rather, they are purely (or blindly) statistical. Many of the questions implicit in the concept of natural weight, for instance, are entirely ignored in the calculation of these values. The charts of ideal weights ask simply, How much do you weigh? Are you above the acceptable range for your sex, age, and height? The implication is that an affirmative answer to the second question spells danger. Left unasked are subtler questions, which we could phrase as, "Am I heavy or light compared to my *natural* weight? Does my pattern of recent weight increases or decreases affect my mortality risk? What if reaching my ideal weight entails activating the defenses against change discussed in the previous chapter?" In short, the weight charts do not take into account the notion of natural (as opposed to ideal) weight, nor the defenses of natural weight that counteract our attempts to stray from it. As a result, mortality studies have, in their turn, focused on how fat (or overweight or underweight) a person is, rather than where that person stands relative to his or her natural weight. The conclusions from such studies corroborate the charts in that they specify the weights that minimize risk. What is missing is an assessment of whether, hidden in these statistics, there may be indications of greater or lesser risk when natural weight is considered, and indications that it is not only where you are on the scale that counts, but where you have been. Let us look at some of this research in detail.

A typical conclusion of the medical research on the consequences of being fat is that "overweight may decrease longevity, it may aggravate the onset and clinical progression of other diseases, and it may modify the quality of life associated with one's social or economic status" (Bray, 1976, p. 215). Such conclusions are derived from an overview of a wide variety of studies, large and small, ancient and still in progress, of various samples of people. Such conclusions are also broad generalizations that often fail to do justice to the complexities of the research findings, many, if not most, of which are not all that clear-cut.

The variety of health problems attributed to overweight or obesity is truly staggering. (We must note the distinction between "overweight" and "obesity," which is often blurred. Obesity is a term generally reserved for a condition of extreme overweight; overweight, obviously, covers the ground between "normal" and "obese." Needless to say, there is no generally accepted dividing line between these categories, which is perhaps just as well. Also needless to say, the terms "normal," "overweight," and "obese" usually refer to one's weight relative to actuarial "ideal" weight—not relative to natural weight. Obviously, our contention is that a person could well be actuarially "overweight" and yet at the same time "normal" with reference to his or her natural weight.) Among the ailments alleged to be associated with obesity are coronary heart disease, cerebrovascular disease and stroke, hypertension, plasma lipid disorders (including hypercholesterolemia), diabetes mellitus, gallbladder disease, cardiopulmonary failure, the Pickwickian (obesity–hypoventilation) syndrome, digestive disorders, respiratory insufficiency, cardiac enlargement, liver damage, increased risks from surgery and pregnancy, greater susceptibility to toxicity from anesthetics, sudden death (presumably from myocardial infarction, that is, massive heart attack), skin disorders, kidney problems, hyperinsulinemia and insulin resistance, hyperuricemia (gout), accelerated wear and deterioration of joint surfaces, and accidents (e.g., Angel and Roncari, 1978; Bray, 1976; Drenick, 1979; Mann, 1974). (Perhaps surprisingly, the obese have a lower than average suicide rate [Ron-

59

cari, 1978]; one can only speculate as to the reason. Maybe there's no need for overt suicidal action when such a fearsome array of medical catastrophes is threatening to do the job anyway.)

GENERAL MORTALITY RISKS

A general elevation in mortality has been ascribed to overweight. A Metropolitan Life Insurance study, for instance, compared overweight policyholders with an otherwise similar population of normal weight policyholders (Bray, 1976). Over a 25-year period, overweight individuals had an increased risk of mortality of roughly 50 percent. Another actuarial study found that insured men weighing over 254 pounds had a two-thirds higher mortality risk than normal. The fact that these particular overweight individuals qualified for insurance at all may reflect their being a relatively healthy segment of the overweight population. It is thus conceivable that the excess mortality risk in random comparison of overweights to normals would be even higher.

In these and similar studies, the extent of increased mortality was especially marked in the grossly (at least 40 percent above normal) obese (Drenick, 1979). In fact, a close examination of these studies indicates that in individuals less than 30 percent overweight, there was no significant increase in mortality risk (Bray, 1976). Blanket comparisons of overweights and normals, then, may both reveal and obscure the truth of the matter. If the overweight sample includes a substantial number of high risk (more than 40 percent overweight) cases, then that sample as a whole may be identified as endangered, despite the fact that the mildly overweight may be virtually indistinguishable from normal in terms of mortality risk. Thus, categorizing the mildly and severely overweight together, in one undifferentiated "overweight" category, may seriously overestimate the threat to the mildly overweight.

The foregoing analysis, urging the separate consideration of the mildly and severely overweight, and suggesting that dramatic life-saving interventions may be unnecessary for the mildly overweight—indeed, that any intervention at all might not really be worth it—usually elicits a response of "What can it hurt? Overweight—even mild overweight—is overweight, which is worse than ideal. It can't hurt to get down to normal (or a little below), can it?" As we shall see, it can hurt. As a result, we believe that the distinction between mild and severe overweight is very important: it marks the boundary between where weight loss interventions are likely to hurt (mild overweight) and where they are likely to help (severe overweight).

The latest Framingham study (a study of an entire community over the years) indicates, predictably, elevated mortality in the most overweight fraction of the population (Sorlie, Gordon, and Kannel, 1980). Moderately overweight people in Framingham, however, seem to die at about the same rate as normal weight or even moderately underweight people. As is underscored by these findings, we must begin to exercise some caution in asserting the health hazards of overweight, as opposed to obesity.

Another finding of the Framingham study is that the thinnest people in the sample were even more seriously at risk than were the fattest. This finding, of course, has stirred up some controversy. One interpretation is that many fatal diseases *cause* weight loss, so that severe thinness is a symptom, rather than a cause, of disease. Another possibility, though, is that severe weight loss *is* a contributor to disease, acting as a strain on our vital functions. We shall examine this hypothesis later. In any case, we should not be too surprised at the discovery of increased mortality at this end of the spectrum; after all, even the notion of "ideal weight" implies that there is a *less-*than-ideal weight, just as there is a more-than-ideal weight. (We have all encountered people who believe that going below "ideal" serves to protect them somehow. For some, it's a precaution against the tendency to gain weight and thus reenter the dangerous above-ideal range. Others reason that if being above a certain weight is bad, then being below it must be good —regardless of the fact that the weight in question is alleged to be "ideal." This sort of thinking, of course, is more than a little absurd; nevertheless, it is quite prevalent in dieters nowadays.) Suffice it to say that both logic and the available medical evidence support the notion that one *can* be too thin.

CORONARY HEART DISEASE (CHD)

Returning to the question of being too fat, we find that most of the increased mortality risk allegedly associated with obesity is presumed to reflect a greater incidence of heart disease. A close examination of the data, however, does not provide a very compelling case against fat. Of five studies published between 1947 and 1974, which sought a post-mortem association between overweight and atherosclerosis (by examining people after death for evidence of atherosclerotic disease), four found little or none (Bray, 1976). Of sixteen large population prospective studies since 1940, only 50 percent found any association at all between overweight and coronary heart diseases (Bray, 1976; Pelkonen et al., 1977). Of those studies that did find some statistical association between overweight and CHD, most found that obesity per se was not a problem; it was only in conjunction with other risk factors (e.g., hypertension, diabetes mellitus, cigarette smoking, elevated serum lipids) that obesity contributed to the risk. Before we exonerate obesity altogether, it should be mentioned that obesity *is* often associated with these other risk factors, such as hypertension or elevated serum lipids. However, two points should be borne in mind: first, uncomplicated obesity does *not* appear to be an independent risk factor for CHD; and, second, as discussed earlier, there is a distinction between mild and serious overweight. Fatness seems likely to threaten your heart only when it is associated with factors that promote the more direct threats.

We have all heard statistics about how many extra miles of blood vessels each additional pound of fat entails, and what a strain on the heart this represents. In fact, however, it is not clear whether extra fat represents a dangerous burden on the circulatory system (Mann, 1974). After all, the heart muscle that must strain so to carry the extra weight is by the same token strengthened by that exercise. The issue boils down to the frequency and pattern of exercise of the heart muscle: there is good (regular, not too violent) and bad (sporadic, "overdone") exercise.

The International Cooperative Study of Cardiovascular Epidemiology (Keys et al., 1972) supports our conclusion that moderate fatness is not a risk to one's heart. In the several groups of men included in this study, there was an increased incidence of CHD in the *most* overweight men, but only when both "hard" and "soft" signs were included. Hard signs include actual death and definite heart attacks, while soft signs include angina pectoris, clinical judgment of definite heart disease, and clinical judgment of possible heart disease. When only the hard signs were considered, there was no significantly increased risk for overweight men. Moreover, if the other risk factors (age, blood pressure, serum cholesterol, smoking) were kept comparable, there were no remaining effects of overweight at all.

OVERWEIGHT AND OVEREATING

We have worked our way toward the conclusion that statistical overweight per se is not a hazard to the circulatory system. Still, there does seem to be a suggestion that the factors that do pose a threat to the circulatory system (hypertension, high lipid levels, and so on) are more likely to be present in overweight people. Is this just an indirect indictment of overweight, or is there some other way of making sense of the complicated, involved-but-not-involved role of fat in heart disease?

Although the issue is complex, we believe that a strong case can be made that *overeating* rather than overweight is the major culprit here. And overeating is something that fat people are more likely to do.

It is crucial to emphasize from the outset that being overweight does not necessarily imply overeating. We tend to assume that all overweight people must be gluttons, but the fact of the matter is that fat people do not need appreciably more calories to maintain their weight than do normal weight people. There is a range of "maintenance" calories—roughly between 1,500 and 3,000 per day—required to maintain a stable weight for most people, depending upon their usual activity levels. Fatter people, despite their usually lower activity levels, may tend toward the higher end of the range, although often they do not even do that. In any case, the differences here are measured in perhaps hundreds of calories, not thousands. And more to the point, both fatter and thinner individuals can and do regulate their weight at relatively stable values when they confine themselves to these maintenance allowances.

We consider overeating, then, not to be a matter of comparison between individuals. If person A can maintain her weight on 2,000 calories, whereas person B requires 2,500 calories to maintain the same weight (or even a higher weight), we do not conclude that B overeats relative to A. In the last chapter, we introduced the notion of overweight relative to one's personal, stable norms (natural weight); now we must introduce an analogous concept (natural weight maintenance eating) to provide a sort of baseline or norm against which to judge true (rather than "statistical") overeating. Overeating can thus be defined as eating more than natural weight maintenance requires. It is, consequently, unnatural eating. And, such eating in excess of natural weight requirements may be more prevalent in the overweight.

In later chapters we shall examine in some detail the processes and problems involved in overeating. For the present, it suffices to note that the association between overweight and overeating is not coincidental. As we shall see, some overeating occurs as a result of dieting and the disruptions it produces in natural eating patterns; and dieting, of course, is a prevalent concern of overweight people. Overeating may also occur in the absence of prior dieting, if stress, emotions, boredom, or other such factors are permitted to determine when one eats and stops eating. This sort of overeating will often produce overweight in someone who is not "naturally" fat. (And this overeating-induced overweight may in turn prod the individual to diet, perhaps further disrupting natural eating patterns.)

Many overweight people, then, are overeaters, for one reason or another. But overeating can be found in normal and thin individuals as well: the characteristic undereat–overeat cycles of dieters and the practice of eating for reasons other than hunger, are abundantly evident in all weight classes. Thus, there is no necessary connection between overeating and over-weight, even though they often tend to go together.

But what is the basis for our concern about overeating, rather than overweight per se? What is the connection of overeating to disease?

OVEREATING AND DISEASE

Though overeating tends to be associated with overweight— which permits one to put the blame on overweight when per-haps it might more accurately be placed on overeating—the two "rival" factors are separable, at least in principle. Since the overweight associated with a high natural weight can be main-tained on a stable caloric intake, we may conclude that an *increasing* caloric intake probably involves overeating in our sense of the term. One researcher has noted that serum lipids rise with increasing caloric intake. Similarly, cardiovascular disease shows a stronger relation to weight *gain* (presumptive overeating) than to stable obesity (Mann, 1974). This relation, furthermore, is exaggerated in people whose weight yo-yos repeatedly, as is the case in diet–overeat cycles.

Researchers generally examine people's health simply as a function of their current weight (or percentage overweight). However, if weight *gain* is the problem, it should be more fruitful to look at health as a function of weight change (espe-cially gain) once adulthood is reached. After the onset of adulthood, further weight gain is likely to be "unnatural." (Of course, we all tend to put on a few pounds with the passage of the years; such gradual gains may be quite natural. But we can still ask whether those who gain a lot are less healthy than those who gain only a smaller, "natural" amount.) One study (Heyden et al., 1971) found that weight gain after the age of 20 was more closely related to the incidence of cerebrovascular incidents (strokes) than was weight at age 20. Though neither weight at age 20 or weight gain thereafter predicted heart disease in this study, a report from the Framingham study (Kannel et al., 1967) found angina pectoris and sudden death —though not myocardial infarction—to be related to weight gain as well as to weight.

A study (Abraham, Collins, and Nordsieck, 1971) which examined childhood weight as a predictor of adult morbidity found that *underweight* children were more likely to encounter hypertensive vascular disease as adults. Overweight adults were found to have more hypertension and cardiovascular renal disease—but it turned out that it was *overweight adults who had been underweight children* who were responsible for this effect. The greatest incidence of hypertension, though, was in normal weight adults who had been underweight as children. Most significantly, "Adults who were overweight as *both* children and adults experienced prevalence rates for hypertensive vascular disease comparable to adults who were *average* weight as both children and adults" (p. 282, italics ours).

We are thus drawn to the somewhat radical conclusion that it is not overweight per se that is the problem so much as overeating. An overweight adult who was an overweight child may well be at or near his or her natural weight; and maintenance of even a relatively high natural weight does not require —in fact, cannot tolerate—overeating. By contrast, a low natural weight is more likely to obtain in someone who was *not* overweight as a child; if that person becomes overweight as an adult, the chances are good that overeating may have pushed that person above natural weight. Even normal weight adults who were underweight as children appear to be endangered, presumably because they are above their natural (very low) weight, probably owing to overeating.

Research on fat cell size and number has assumed that it is fat cell number that is most directly indicative of natural weight. As we noted in chapter 2, fat cell number probably does not directly determine natural weight; however, it seems to be a significant correlate of it. In any case, some research has indicated that fat cell number is unrelated to atherosclerosis (Bjurlf, 1959), suggesting that whether one's natural weight is high or low doesn't matter all that much. What *was* found to be related to atherosclerosis was fat cell size, which is usually taken as an indication of whether one is above, below, or at one's natural weight. People with "fatter" fat cells were at higher risk; and these are the people in whom overeating (i.e., eating more than natural weight maintenance requires) is most likely.

Whether one is 30 pounds (or even 30 percent) overweight, then, seems to us not quite the right question to ask when assessing health concerns. Rather, we are inclined to ask whether that degree of overweight is attributable to overeating. There are two problem scenarios here: first, the person with a high natural weight who diets and becomes involved in repeated loss–gain cycles, with much of the gaining due to overeating (not just gradual regaining on a moderate, sensible, regulated diet); and, second, the person with a low or average natural weight whose weight is nevertheless driven above its natural level by overeating, for whatever emotional or "dynamic" reason. These are pure cases. Others are identifiable, such as the person with an average natural weight who decides to diet anyway, in a quest for absolute thinness. In this case, the person may become trapped in a diet–overeat cycle despite not having been overweight in the first place (except relative to a personal, unrealistic standard probably derived from the media). What characterizes all these cases is the presence of unnatural, excessive eating beyond the requirements for maintaining one's natural weight. It is to such excess that nature appears to take exception, in the form of life-threatening disease.

HYPERTENSION

We have mentioned hypertension (high blood pressure) in passing, as one of the serious risk factors often attributed to overweight. A closer examination of the evidence suggests some of the complexities involved in trying to determine causality, risk, and blame. We must begin by acknowledging that most studies do find an increased incidence of hypertension in the overweight (Bray, 1976). (For a while, there was some concern that this association might be spurious, an artifact of the way blood pressure is measured. The thickness of one's arm can affect the readings, especially if a "short" cuff type sphygmomanometer is used.) In any case, many recent studies have found a marked association between blood pressure and weight, with overweight persons showing up to twice as much hypertension as normals (and three times the incidence for their underweight counterparts) (Bray, 1976; Stambi et al.,

1978). A recent review concluded that for every 10 kilogram (22 pound) increase in weight, baseline systolic blood pressure rises 3mm, and diastolic rises 2mm (Drenick, 1979).

The foregoing conclusions, however, were qualified: it seems that the relation between more weight and higher blood pressure is *especially* true for *adult* onset obesity—and this is the sort of excessive weight gain that we suspect may represent overeating rather than a high natural weight per se.

Evidence provided by studies indicating that weight loss usually leads to a reduction in blood pressure (Angel and Roncari, 1978; Bray, 1976; Heyden et al., 1971) is open to several interpretations. One inference might be simply that overweight causes hypertension, so that the removal of the cause (overweight) likewise removes the effect (hypertension). Alternatively, it may be that being above one's *natural* weight is the cause, as is suggested by the studies comparing childhood and adult fatness. Finally, it might not be the weight so much as the overeating—which produces the higher-than-natural weight—that is to blame. Weight loss demands the cessation of overeating, and this perhaps is the value of losing weight. These alternatives are obviously difficult to disentangle—but they should alert us yet again to the fact that a "simple" association between overweight and a health risk is often subject to various interpretations, and that we should not necessarily jump to the most obvious conclusion.

DIABETES

Like hypertension, diabetes on first glance appears to be clearly related to overweight (Angel and Roncari, 1978; Bray, 1976; Drenick, 1979), because of an increased strain on the pancreas. Closer examination of the data, however, reveals that insulin resistance and diabetes in overweight people are attributable more to overeating than to overweight (Angel and Roncari, 1978). This in fact makes some intuitive sense: since it is eating that calls forth insulin from the pancreas, overeating seems the more likely pancreatic stressor.

Again as with hypertension, it appears to be the case that adult onset obesity—which we have argued is largely a matter of overeating—is most dangerous in promoting diabetes. One Veterans Administration study found that more than half of a sample of grossly obese who had been overweight for an average of 25 years had diabetes mellitus. But at the age of 18 (or older), none of these men had been fat or diabetic; all had passed their armed forces physicals. Thus, it is adult onset obesity on which we can blame this startling incidence of diabetes. (Of course, it has been argued that it is diabetes that causes obesity, and not vice versa; in either case, it does not seem to be overweight per se that is the problem.)

In another study (Drenick, 1979), a group of nondiabetic men with long-standing obesity reduced their weight to normal levels; most quickly regained this lost weight. Within 6 years, 80 percent of the men had developed impaired glucose tolerance and were considered diabetic or at risk for diabetes. This study suggests strongly that weight fluctuations—especially gains—are more conducive to the development of diabetes than is overweight alone.

SERUM LIPIDS

Elevated levels of serum lipids (e.g., cholesterol, triglyceride, free fatty acids) have been found in overweight individuals

(Angel and Roncari, 1978; Bray, 1976; Drenick, 1979) and are considered a serious health risk. In the case of cholesterol, however, weight loss by dieting appears to have only a transitory beneficial effect, since the decline in cholesterol values during weight loss is not maintained once a stable lower weight is reached. It seems that it is not weighing less but eating less that helps. Similarly, although high triglyceride levels are common in the obese, normal and even low values are frequently seen (Drenick, 1979). More pertinent is the finding of an association between overweight and high triglyceride levels only in patients who gained weight after age 20–25 (Bray, 1976). This statistic meshes nicely with the finding that triglyceride levels are related to the carbohydrate content of one's diet. As we mentioned earlier, Mann (1974) found that serum lipids rise with increasing caloric intake, not weight per se; Rogers et al. (1980) likewise found no relation between weight per se and serum lipids.

In one of our studies (Hibscher and Herman, 1977), we found that there was a modest correlation between the extent of overweight and free fatty acid levels. However, this correlation was misleading in the sense that overweight subjects were much more likely to be dieters, and it was dieters (fat, thin, or normal weight) who showed high FFA levels. Once again, the culprit seems to be weight change—gaining weight, dieting, or yo-yoing—or deviation from one's natural weight, rather than excess weight according to the actuarial ideal.

GALL BLADDER DISEASE

Theoretically, obesity causes gallstones by causing elevated cholesterol in the bile. Excess cholesterol tends to crystallize and result in gallstone formation (Angel and Roncari, 1978; Bray, 1976). The relation between cholesterol and overweight, however, is complex, so we must be cautious in interpreting the statistics "demonstrating" increased gall bladder disease as a function of overweight, with 30–35 percent of "morbidly" obese adults having gallstones (e.g., Angel and Roncari, 1978; Drenick, 1979). There seems to be as much evidence that weight loss promotes gallstone formation as that weight gain is the problem (Roncari, 1978). And both loss and gain seem to be more problematic for cholesterol than is weight stability.

CONCLUSIONS

Our analysis of the various disorders supposedly caused by overweight makes it difficult to accept blindly the notion that there is an ideal weight that minimizes the risk of disease. Actuarially defined overweight is confounded in much of the relevant research with what we are calling true overweight (i.e., above-natural weight). And both are confounded to a large extent with true overeating. A sober analysis of the facts does not support the notion that a particular degree of moderate overweight is necessarily dangerous. Even relatively large amounts of fat may pose no serious threat, though the data are less clear on this point. What does seem to create problems are the wild weight swings often seen in overweight dieters. These swings almost inevitably involve bouts of overeating alternating with stretches of relative abstinence. And the end result, as we'll discuss in detail later, may be that the overweight dieter, by disengaging his eating from its natural regulatory controls, ends up overweight not only by actuarial standards but even by his own physiological (natural weight) standards. This, we believe, is the sort of overweight that is to be avoided.

Being fat may in and of itself pose some medical problems. Surgery is often more difficult and dangerous, as is pregnancy. One's joints may suffer from the strain of weight. A less obvious consequence of fatness is that it seems to discourage people from seeking medical treatment (Drenick, 1979), possibly because doctors who treat overweight patients tend to see them as weak-willed, awkward, and generally less worthy of their attention (Bray, 1976). Fat people's reluctance to see doctors —or have doctors see them—may result in their receiving diagnoses and treatment later on in the course of their illnesses than normals; their diseases may have more opportunity to progress to the point of inflicting severe damage.

If doctors react negatively to fatness, it is the patients who suffer. But it is the doctors who are to blame. As we have seen, the medical indictment of fatness (defined relative to the charts on doctors' office walls) is largely based on an incomplete analysis of what is causing what. To the extent that the medical community directly or indirectly encourages radical weight loss attempts without reference to one's natural weight history and without regard to the bad eating habits (including overeating) that ensue, it may be doing as much harm as good.

CHAPTER 4

Dangers of Dieting

WE HAVE SUGGESTED that being overweight in and of itself may not be as serious a medical threat as has often been alleged. If one's weight is relatively high but also relatively stable, there may be little reason—at least, little medical reason—for concern. If one has driven one's weight above one's natural weight by chronic overeating, then it seems that perhaps one might truly regard one's weight as excessive and weight loss as worthwhile. Yet, even in this case, what makes weight loss a medically commendable goal is probably the fact that weight loss techniques ordinarily preclude overeating. For someone who does not overeat, and who is not involved in repeated gain–loss cycles, the value of weight loss is less clear.

Still, there are other concerns in life besides health, and one may have other motives for attempting to lose weight, as we shall see in subsequent chapters. Even if being statistically overweight is not in and of itself unhealthy, cannot one choose to reject overweight on other grounds? Besides, isn't it healthier in general to lose weight? As might be anticipated from our previous discussions, the answer is a qualified *no*.

As we have seen, the defense of natural weight is designed to counteract our attempts to shift our weight too radically from its naturally regulated levels. The defenses themselves are geared toward restoring natural weight, but if these defenses are overrun, as may occur in the case of the truly determined dieter, then illness may ensue. After all, as we've suggested, one's natural weight is not defended frivolously; it is defended because of its biological value. Illness is the result of violating biological norms. We might thus expect weight loss in violation of natural weight norms to pose medical problems.

Still, we've also emphasized the fact that many overweight people may well be maintaining (or increasing) a weight above biological norms. Indeed, in the last chapter we attributed some fairly serious diseases to being above one's natural weight, or at least to the overeating responsible for one's weight rising to that unnaturally high level. Accordingly, we should expect that weight loss directed at lowering one's weight from an unnaturally high level down to a more moderate, natural level would meet with little biological resistance, and pose correspondingly little threat to one's health. In general, we believe that such weight loss is indeed desirable for medical reasons, not to mention other reasons that may pertain.

However, the distinction between "bad" weight loss (i.e., down below natural weight) and "good" weight loss (i.e., down to natural weight) may be too simple to capture all the complexities implied by weight regulation. For instance, the long-term regulation of weight is probably not the only homeostatic process of relevance to the issue of weight loss. Short-term regulation must also be considered, as the immediate metabolic needs of our bodies also demand attention. Although the hugely overweight individual, who may be well above set point, can presumably afford to lose dozens or scores of pounds, the *manner* and *rate* of weight loss may affect his or her health, independently of the overall value of weight loss. Dramatic feats of dieting or fasting may produce weight losses which, while perfectly acceptable in terms of general, long-term weight regulation, may nonetheless threaten the individual's well-being in terms of short-term, specific nutritional requirements. To put matters bluntly, even "good," healthy weight loss may be achieved through "bad," dangerous dietary practices.

WEIGHT LOSS AND REGULATION

It is a common observation that many people who lose weight eventually regain it, often with interest. This observation is consistent with our analysis of natural weight regulation (see chapter 2), since it implies that people who drop below their natural weights will eventually find that the lost weight is "restored," either through eating or through metabolic adjustments. The metabolic adjustments, in fact, may provide the "interest" which more than compensates for the weight lost originally.

Another problem facing the individual attempting to drop below his or her natural weight is that this ambition almost necessarily entails developing some way of ignoring or otherwise avoiding the blandishments of hunger cues; these directive signals are naturally augmented in the person whose weight drops below its biologically appropriate value. Bombarded by such signals, the dieter must overcome them, either by learning to misperceive them or to not perceive them at all or by adopting a radical diet (such as some fasts) that apparently eliminates the signals. Although these tactics are often successful for the immediate purpose of weight loss, they are ultimately counterproductive. If one develops the habit of not responding to hunger cues during one's diet, one will almost certainly have trouble responding to them later on, when one wishes simply to maintain a lower weight. The problem facing the successful weight loser becomes, "If I cannot rely on hunger cues as a guide for eating, on what *can* I rely?" The answer almost inevitably involves some artificial guides, divorced from one's genuine regulatory needs. (Indeed, if the diet succeeds in reducing weight below its natural level, attention to one's genuine regulatory needs would produce weight gain.) Likewise, satiety cues appear to be linked, in a form of regulatory opposition, to hunger cues, so that successful dieting produces a loss of access to guides for stopping eating as well as to those for starting. As we shall see in subsequent chapters, dependence on the mental guidelines that dieters tend to substitute for natural hunger–satiety signals is very risky. Such dependence is subject to all sorts of disruptions and "exceptions," which in turn can produce serious overeating (along with alternating undereating). Individuals who diet themselves down below their natural weights, then, risk rapid relapse; and the relapse often occurs without the natural brake of satiety signals that might otherwise inhibit overeating, since such signals had to be jettisoned, along with the attached hunger signals, in order for one to succeed at losing weight in the first place.

Dangers of Dieting

Dieting below one's natural weight, then, poses risks in terms of possible loss of touch with one's regulatory checks and balances. But what about dieting *toward* one's natural weight if one starts out from above? What is the danger here? The danger is precisely the same: namely, that one will lose access to one's normal regulatory signals, with the result that even when one has been restored to one's natural weight, one will be dependent on artificial and unreliable guides for eating and not eating.

There is nothing about lowering one's weight from a level above natural weight that demands that one ignore or deny the regulatory signals of hunger and satiety. After all, our previous analysis suggests that in this situation the defense of natural weight will operate so as to make eating in accordance with those signals weight reducing. Why, then, does such weight loss so often proceed *without* any connection to normal defensive regulatory signals? There are two basic reasons for this "perversity." First, many people—probably most people—who achieve a weight above their natural level do so by *overcoming* normal defensive regulatory signals; the very fact that they are above natural levels suggests that they have already become unresponsive to these signals—or perhaps that they never were responsive to them, for whatever reason of faulty conditioning or perceptual learning. Thus, losing weight naturally is an option that is essentially closed to them, unless they can somehow "reconnect" with their regulatory signals. (We shall discuss in our final chapter how this "reconnection" might be accomplished.)

The second reason for the "perverse" inability of people above their natural weights to lose weight naturally is sheer impatience. In a culture where "miracle" diets are supposedly capable of ridding one of 10 or 20 pounds in a week, the natural restorative process is often insufficiently quick or dramatic to suit the dieter's ambition. While reliance on natural hunger and satiety cues might do the job effectively and permanently, the temptation to do the job quickly is simply too attractive. (And besides, as we shall see, reliance on natural hunger and satiety cues doesn't sound, to most prospective dieters, as if it will work.) Adoption of quick weight loss techniques, of course, involves overriding natural signals—even though those signals are pointing in the same direction—in order to get there faster. The result is that one reaches one's weight loss goal more rapidly, but without one's natural regulatory processes synchronized to behavior. One has returned to natural weight, but the speed of the return and the insensitive manner in which it was accomplished jeopardize one's chances of remaining there comfortably.

DIRECT RISKS OF WEIGHT LOSS

One problem with losing weight unnaturally and/or dissociating oneself from the natural regulators of body weight is that, as we have seen, such weight loss is precariously maintained and likely to be disrupted. When weight gain eventually occurs, as it probably will, it is likely to involve the sort of medically dangerous overeating that we examined (and castigated) in the last chapter. However, precipitate and unnatural weight gain is not the only charge that can be brought against weight loss.

Medical disorders that have been attributed directly to weight loss (independent of subsequent weight gain and/or yo-yoing) include the following: hypotension (low blood pressure) and fainting, elevated serum cholesterol and gallstones, diarrhea, aching muscles, general weakness and fatigue, both bradycardia (slowed heart rate) and increased heart rate, changes in head hair (becoming thin, sparse, and red tinged), abdominal pains, elevated uric acid levels (which can lead to gout or kidney stones), anemia, gouty arthritis, edema, headache, nausea, cardiac disorders, and even death from various complications (Angel and Roncari, 1978; Baird, Parsons, and Howard, 1974; Bray, 1976; Drenick et al., 1964; Duncan et al., 1964, 1965; Garnett et al., 1969; Jung et al., 1979; Kannel and Gordon, 1974; Kark, Johnson, and Lewis, 1945; Kollar and Atkinson, 1966; Landsberg and Young, 1978; Marliss, 1978; Rooth and Carlstrom, 1970; Stunkard and McLaren-Hume, 1959). These disorders are complex and often interrelated; moreover, it is often difficult to determine precisely what aspect of dieting (e.g., speed, severity, specific nutritional deficits) is responsible for any particular symptom. Some dieters experience few if any symptoms and most of the commonly experienced symptoms are relatively unproblematic (e.g., low blood pressure and dizziness, fainting, nausea and other gastric distress, weakness and fatigue). The fact remains, however, that even apart from the risks of subsequent overeating, dieting often poses direct dangers to one's health. The specific dangers, of course, depend on the diet.

The following excerpt from a news report in a recent edition of the *Toronto Star* provides a graphic illustration of the hazards of overly zealous weight loss:

A medical expert on nutrition . . . told a coroner's jury that J.C. should have been on a diet, but not the radical one she was trying to adhere to when she suddenly collapsed and died last May. [Dr. M.] testified that Mrs. C. . . . had too many physical and psychological problems to be on a diet that limited her to about 900 calories a day. . . . All 3 medical experts have said they suspect that Mrs. C. died as a result of an . . . irregular heartbeat induced by a combination of the drugs she was taking and her poor physical condition.

In this instance, the dieter was enrolled in a branch of a national weight loss organization, with 11 days remaining in an 18-week diet program for which she had paid $626.40. Her family doctor had seen and approved a description of the diet and other methods used by the clinic. In addition, the doctor had prescribed diuretics (to remove water from the body) and a hunger suppressant for Mrs. C., as well as an antidepressant. (As we shall see in later chapters, dieting and weight loss sometimes precipitate depression.) The combination of insufficient calories and "diet-enhancing" drugs appears to have led to the death of this dieter—and probably countless others. It is ironic that most such deaths are blamed on the victims' overweight rather than the true culprit, radical attempts to lose weight. A major reason that Mrs. C.'s death was investigated so thoroughly and correctly diagnosed was that she died in the lobby of the building housing the weight loss clinic she was attending.

Although deaths such as Mrs. C.'s are clearly the most serious side effects of weight loss attempts, they are by no means the only ones.

PILLS AND OTHER DRUGS

Our culture, for various reasons, is strongly oriented toward pill taking as a problem-solving technique. If overweight is a "disease," then there ought to be some sort of medicine that one can take to correct it. Diet pills are specifically designed to diminish or eliminate one's appetite or hunger, and thus "correct" the overeating that is supposedly responsible for overweight.

There are two interesting flaws in the logic behind the use of appetite suppressants. First, some overweight people are naturally overweight, as we have seen; excessive appetite is not the culprit in their case, since there is little evidence that they eat appreciably more than anyone else. (This is not to say that pill-induced undereating will not produce weight loss, even if only in the short term.) A second logical flaw is that most people who are fat because of overeating (i.e., those who are above their natural weights) overeat precisely because they don't respond appropriately to hunger and satiety cues. Even if diet pills succeeded in eliminating hunger signals altogether, there might be no evident effect on eating, since eating, for these people, depends on so many factors other than hunger. Thus, the basis for our reliance on diet pills is suspect.

Some pills are directed less at eating than at hormonal or metabolic processes implicated in fat storage. Again, there is little evidence that these processes are in any way in need of correction. Although the pills may produce temporary alterations and some short-term weight loss, changes are more likely to be from a normal metabolic situation toward an abnormal or disordered one than vice versa. One drug, dinitrophenol, was popular in the 1950s as a "treatment" for obesity, because it supposedly increased metabolic rate. It was ultimately outlawed because of its extreme toxic effects (Feinstein, 1960). "Hormone pills," typically thyroid preparations, usually have little or no effect beyond interfering with normal hormone production, which can lead to serious complications (Drenick, 1979).

The most popular diet pills have been those in the pharmacological family of amphetamines. Most well-controlled studies have failed to substantiate the claim that amphetamines promote significant or lasting weight loss; certainly they are no more effective than adherence to a moderately calorically restrictive diet. In one study (Stunkard, Rickels, and Hesbacher, 1973), amphetamine users lost an average of only 6 pounds in a 7-week period.

Still, for many people it is easier to swallow a pill than to worry about adhering to a diet, no matter how generous. The cost that must be paid for this short cut, however, is excessive: amphetamines often involve tolerance (which means higher and higher doses) and addiction, psychoticlike episodes from chronic high doses, insomnia, and even death (Bray, 1976).

Fenfluramine, an amphetaminelike diet pill popular in Europe, is alleged to be both less dangerous than the amphetamines and neither addictive nor tolerance inducing. Relatively minor side effects (drowsiness, dizziness, headache, insomnia, and gastrointestinal complaints such as nausea, vomiting, diarrhea, and constipation) are common, however; and fenfluramine seems to be no more effective than amphetamine in inducing long-term weight loss.

Nausea is usually considered, and with good reason, to be an undesirable side effect of diet pills. But because nausea is basically incompatible with eating, it suggests itself as a "diet aid." Thus one group of courageous—albeit foolhardy—dieters took digitalis, a potent cardiac medication that is nausea producing (Feinstein, 1960). They were fortunate not to develop cardiac complications; digitalis combined with amphetamines has been associated with severe complications and even fatalities (Drenick, 1979). Belladonna and apomorphine, two nausea-producing agents which are potentially quite dangerous, have also been tried; fortunately, both were deemed ineffective and abandoned as "diet" drugs (Feinstein, 1960).

One other type of "diet medication" deserves mention. Laxatives and diuretics remain popular as instruments of quick weight loss. Diuretics are quite effective for short-term weight loss; the lost weight, however, is water, not fat, and is regained as soon as the use of diuretics is discontinued (Feinstein, 1960). More serious is the fact that regular use of laxatives and diuretics can result in serious electrolyte imbalances, potassium deficiency, and disregulation of the excretory system; these problems in turn imperil the heart and circulatory system as well as the abdominal and muscular systems. In severe cases, death is a possibility. On balance, none of the perils involved in taking diet "medicines" seems worth the risk—especially since a sensible, calorically restricted diet is likely to be at least as effective.

FAD DIETS

Although sensible dieting is less dangerous and at least as effective as drug-assisted dieting, people seem to shy away from sensible diets. The common sense diets are—relatively speaking—"good for you", but somehow "good for you" has an almost pejorative tone to it. Why be a tortoise when one can be a hare? Why work hard when some "trick" built into the diet "does all the work for you"? Fad diets all promise "miraculous" weight loss accomplishments, usually with little or no effort, because the particular diet constituents are combined so as to "burn off calories" or in some other way take advantage of a metabolic short cut to weight loss. Such diets have some value, but this value is principally a matter of inflated earnings by diet authors and their publishers. Your (repeated) failure to lose is their gain. We shall not examine the most transparently inappropriate of these diets (such as the "banana diet," the "rice diet," or the "hardboiled eggs and grapefruit diet"); these single-food, all-you-can-eat diets obviously would give rise to any number of vitamin and mineral deficiency disorders, if one were able to stay on them long enough to lose a significant amount of weight. Fortunately, few people even attempt to adhere to these diets for more than a few days.

LOW CARBOHYDRATE DIETS

The most popular type of diet over the past couple of decades has been one or another variation on the theme of drastically restricting carbohydrate intake while liberally allowing protein and fat consumption. This type of diet has appeared in many versions, including the *Air Force Diet,* Taller's *Calories Don't Count Diet,* the *Drinking Man's Diet,* and Stillman's *Doctor's Quick Weight Loss Diet;* its most recent incarnation has been Atkins's *Diet Revolution.* The hazards of such diets are now reasonably well known: much of the large initial weight loss experienced is water loss, and dehydration can result if the water is not replaced; sodium depletion is also a potential problem; and very high protein intake strains the kidneys. Other risks include hyperlipidemia (high blood lipid levels), implicated, as we saw, in coronary heart disease; acceleration of atherosclerosis; elevated uric acid levels in the blood, promoting gout; postural hypotension, a drop in blood pressure when moving from a prone to an upright position; and various minor problems like fatigue and listlessness. Atkins claims that his diet releases a "fat mobilizing hormone," but the existence of such a hormone has yet to be clearly demonstrated.

A graphic illustration of the hazards of low carbohydrate diets was inadvertently provided by the Canadian Army (Kark, Johnson, and Lewis, 1945), which was experimenting with pemmican (dried meat consisting of approximately 70 percent fat and 30 percent protein) as an emergency ration for soldiers. Soldiers given unlimited amounts of nothing but pemmican and tea were incapacitated *within 3 days* and "the platoon [was at] the point of disintegration as a military unit" (p. 346). The men were dizzy, nauseous to the point of vomiting, highly susceptible to cold temperatures, exhausted, dehydrated, and listless; they showed neurological changes and a very low level of physical fitness. They were diagnosed as suffering from caloric deficiency with ketosis, dehydration, salt depletion, and ascorbic acid depletion. The officers commanding this unit agreed that if they had actually been involved in combat, they would all have been casualties by their second day on pemmican. If soldiers in top physical condition respond so alarmingly to such a carbohydrate free diet, one can only wonder about its effects on average, out-of-shape dieters. Even with carbohydrate added to a low calorie protein diet, hospitalized patients developed complications like bradycardia, diarrhea, hair loss and discoloration, colicky abdominal pains, elevated serum cholesterol, and asymptomatic anemia (Baird, Parsons, and Howard, 1974).

In its evaluation of low carbohydrate diets, the American Medical Association Council on Foods and Nutrition (1973) concludes: "If such diets are truly successful, why then do they fade into obscurity within a relatively short period only to be resurrected some years later in slightly different guise? Moreover, despite the claims of universal and painless success for such diets, no nationwide decrease in obesity has been reported" (p. 1415). It bears repeating that such diets are not simply ineffective; were that the case, dieters' cyclical crazes would merely provide the basis for cynical remarks on the folly of human nature. These diets are more than fashions, even though they are currently treated as such. They are positively dangerous, and should be appreciated as a significant threat to health.

FASTING AND ITS MODIFICATIONS

Since most dieters are eventually forced to the conclusion that the only way to lose weight is by dramatic caloric reduction, many eventually experiment with fasting. This may mean eliminating caloric intake altogether, or, as in the liquid protein diet, ingesting the minimum amount of protein necessary to stave off excess nitrogen loss and prevent the breakdown of protein in muscle and organ tissue. Such fasting does in fact produce substantial and relatively rapid weight loss, and often has the additional advantage of producing loss of appetite during the period of starvation. It is also easier for many people to avoid real food altogether than to be constrained to too little. The question that remains, though, is, how healthy is fasting? How does it compare to not losing at all?

On the plus side, when these fasts are undertaken with close medical supervision, benefits may include reduction of blood pressure to normal ranges in hypertensive patients, normalization of blood glucose levels in maturity onset diabetics not using insulin, and decreased insulin requirements in diabetics on insulin. Furthermore, individuals who actually lose large amounts of weight show improved effort tolerance, decreased symptoms from hiatus hernias, and improvement in symptoms due to osteoarthritis of the back, hips, and knees (Marliss, 1978). In some respects, then, the use of short-term, protein-sparing modified fasts may be considered successful for patients treated in a hospital with an individually tailored diet of high quality protein (Bistrian and Sherman, 1978; Bistrian et al., 1977). However, for the vast majority of potential dieters, personal hospitalized treatment is neither feasible nor justified. Thousands, perhaps millions, of people thus turned to liquid protein "supplements" to institute their own protein-sparing modified fasts or "last chance" diets.

Examination of the negative effects of these modified fasts does not leave much doubt as to whether the likely risks outweigh the likely benefits. The fluid and electrolyte shifts in the first week to 10 days which cause the initial rapid weight loss also lead to postural hypotension and increased pulse rate. A concurrent depletion in the body's potassium level is possible, causing fatigue, muscle weakness, and cardiac arhythmias. The long-term use of very low calorie protein diets can result in calcium, mineral, and trace metal deficits, the full range of complications from which are not yet fully understood (Marliss, 1978). As with the low carbohydrate diets, protein-supplemented fasts lead to high levels of uric acid in the blood (by the same mechanism which reduces one's appetite), which can lead to gout, kidney stones, nausea and/or vomiting, and changes in liver functioning. Gastrointestinal effects include constipation and the associated risk of impacted feces (also common on whole protein diets) or diarrhea (more common with hydrolyzed protein). Endocrine function is altered, possibly causing a relatively hypothyroid state which may explain other frequent side effects like lowered basal metabolic rate, cold intolerance, dry skin, hair loss, and muscle cramps. Amenorrhea in women and decreased libido in both sexes may also occur (Marliss, 1978). Finally, as of 1978, the United States Food and Drug Administration had received reports of no less than fifty deaths associated with very low calorie diet use. At least fifteen of these deaths occurred in women aged 25 to 51 without known predisposing problems, twelve of whom were under a doctor's care. It is clear—or should be—that fasting, modified or not, may well be one's "last chance," but not necessarily for the reasons suggested by its advocates.

A person who is willing to risk whatever side effects appear while on these regimens will face even more problems after the desired amount of weight has been lost. Upon reaching the target weight, the dieter must begin to eat more normal amounts of food (calories) and varieties of nutrients, especially carbohydrates. This process, known as "refeeding," entails risks of its own. For example, there are likely to be fluid and electrolyte shifts opposite to those that occurred at the beginning of the diet; during refeeding, fluid retention occurs and may even cause edema (swelling). Weight increases, owing to the fluid retention, even if actual caloric intake is still below the body's requirements; and, if too much water is retained, sodium, chloride, and especially potassium deficiencies may result, unless supplements are added to the normal food intake (Marliss, 1978). Even more serious, and possibly fatal, are biliary tract disorders (e.g., gallbladder "attacks") and pancreatic complications. Four of the deaths associated with the protein diet occurred during refeeding—including two from pancreatitis and one involving a perforated stomach (Marliss, 1978).

Considering the hazards of protein-supplemented fasts, we would expect to find ample agreement as to the comparable or even greater dangers of nonsupplemented, total fasts. Surprisingly, though, there is some support in the medical literature for true fasting as a weight loss technique. Both short-term (often repeated intermittently) and long-term fasts have been advocated. Short-term fasts, of 2 weeks or less, are favored by several researchers because of their effectiveness in inducing weight loss and their lack of serious side effects. The earliest modern report of short-term fasting as a treatment for obesity (Bloom, 1959) claimed that in 4–9 day fasts, overweight patients experienced nothing more severe than mild headaches or epigastric distress and were not even intensely hungry. A later report advocating repeated short-term fasts (Duncan et al., 1964) claimed that only one of fourteen patients suffering from gout had an attack brought on by fasting; other symptoms such as weakness, nausea, dizziness, and headaches were seen as minor compared to the beneficial effects experienced by patients suffering from hypertension, diabetes, angina, chronic myocardial insufficiency, emphysema, and psoriasis. Two patients with chronic cardiovascular disease suffered transient attacks of auricular flutter when they violated the authors' "anti-exercise rule" and walked 2–6 miles a day. But the authors concluded that brief periods of fasting are tolerated well by obese subjects, cause clinical improvement, and seem advisable for overweight patients who are not pregnant and do not suffer from uncontrolled labile diabetes, progressive diabetic neuropathy, recent coronary infarction, or any kind of acute infection or hepatic disease. A subsequent report on 900 obese patients from the same investigative team (Duncan et al., 1965) reiterated the favorable effects of fasting on preexisting disorders but modified the recommendation for brief repeated fasts to include only severely obese patients who have been unable to reduce using "conventional" methods, who have no contraindication to fasting, and whose physical activity is restricted to a minimum. Thus, even researchers who advocate short-term fasting seem to feel that it should only be attempted in a hospital setting (Duncan et al., 1965; Gilliland, 1968; Harrison and Harden, 1966) and that there are likely to be side effects including nausea and vomiting, weakness or dizziness, and headaches or muscle cramps (Genuth, Castro, and Vestes, 1974). Furthermore, there is a lack of agreement with respect to the long-term benefits of this weight loss procedure. Some reports claim that most patients remain at a lower weight (Bloom, 1959) but, in general, reports have indicated that 31 (Duncan et al., 1964) to 55 (Genuth et al., 1978) percent of the patients return to their original weight *or higher* within a year or two.

Given the high "relapse" rates and the frequent side effects as reported above—plus more serious ones, such as loss of lean body tissue, edema, and tachycardia (Ball, Canary, and Kyle, 1967; Herman and Iverson, 1968)—many other researchers conclude that short-term fasting is stressful for the patient and may not be the treatment of choice for obesity.

When we consider these negative reports on short-term fasts, we should not be surprised to discover even more serious problems frequently associated with long-term fasts. In addition to a dramatic rise in emotional complications (Stunkard and Rush, 1974), which will be discussed in more detail in the next chapter, fasts lasting more than 2 weeks are often found to cause side effects such as atrophy of the villi in the small intestine, serious edema, parotitis (infection of the saliva-producing parotid gland), a myocardial ischemic episode, breakdown in electrolyte homeostasis, severe hypotension, severe anemia and gout arthritis, changes in number and shape of white blood cells, severe cardiovascular complications, hypokalemia (potassium deficiency), gout, and death from various causes (Cubberley, Polster, and Schulman, 1965; Drenick and Alvarez, 1971; Drenick et al., 1964; Garnett et al., 1969; Kollar and Atkinson, 1966; Munro et al., 1970; Rooth and Carlstrom, 1970; Runcie and Thomson, 1970; Sandhofer et al., 1973; Spencer, 1968; Thomson, Runcie and Miller, 1966). Since there seems to be at least a 50 percent chance that the weight lost by fasting will be regained (Bray, 1976) and since the serious complications and deaths occurred despite hospitalization and careful monitoring of pertinent body functions, long-term fasting seems to be at least as potentially harmful as the overweight problem it is meant to alleviate.

BYPASSES

Because fasting—like most other forms of dieting—ultimately depends on the dieter's ability or motivation to resist temptation, it is never a foolproof approach. Cheating—or, as the professionals call it, "noncompliance"—is always a threat to the success of the diet or fast; and many, if not most, dieters have a well-developed image of themselves as unable to resist temptation to the extent necessary to achieve success. This view is widely shared by the medical profession. It is not surprising that both doctors and patients are attracted by the possibility of "surgical dieting," or bypass operations. These operations are designed, basically, to reduce the digestive tract's capacity to absorb food; thus, regardless of how much the dieter feels like eating, there will be an inescapable upper limit on how many calories can be absorbed and metabolized. Will power should no longer be an issue.

93

The earliest attempts to bypass part of the intestine, in the 1960s, were not particularly successful, at least when the risks were subtracted from the benefits. Severe electrolyte losses and liver failure were common; seventeen of the seventy patients treated died (Bray, 1976).

The first sort of bypass procedure was soon superseded by the jejunoileostomy, which is the intestinal bypass operation in use today. Only patients 100 or more pounds above their (actuarial) ideal weight are eligible for this radical treatment, because the risks remain considerable. The benefits, however, are often dramatic: patients tend to lose about one-third of their weight, and keep it off; cholesterol and triglyceride levels are reduced along with blood pressure; joint functioning improves; and diabetics experience a lessened need for insulin.

The experience of those who have had the operation—even the most successful cases—has not been exactly what was initially anticipated, however. For one thing, the expectation that the patients could eat as much as they wanted was soon dashed; diarrhea, hemorrhoids, and related side effects soon constrained food intake to smaller proportions, if only to minimize discomfort. Patients ended up eating much less, which may account for the beneficial effects on cholesterol, triglyceride, and blood pressure levels.

If diarrhea were the only problem of intestinal bypass operations, they would probably be more popular than they are. (One recent best-selling diet "authority," the author of the Beverly Hills diet, has argued that the more time spent in the bathroom, the better.) Diarrhea is almost universal, but it is by no means the most serious risk involved. Other side effects include pulmonary emboli (blood clots in the lungs), gastrointestinal hemorrhage, kidney failure, electrolyte imbalance, liver disease, urinary tract stones, anemia, assorted other intestinal problems, and wound infection from the operation itself. If a patient later becomes pregnant, her child may be born mentally retarded as a result of prenatal malnutrition. Finally, there is a nontrivial risk of death even in the safer medical environments; and, for some of the less well-conducted series of operations, mortality rates have run as high as 5 or 10 percent.

The same risks appear to apply to a newer procedure, which involves closing off part of the stomach, rather than the intestine. Overall, the side effects of this type of operation tend to be less pronounced than with intestinal bypass—but a death rate of approximately 3 percent is not to be trifled with.

Given such consequences, some writers have questioned whether bypass operations should be performed except in truly extreme circumstances. Wooley et al. (1980) have pointed out that if an effective antiobesity drug were found "it would be many years before it would be available to the public and if its mortality and morbidity risks were comparable to those of gastric and intestinal bypass it seems doubtful that its use would ever be approved" (p. 470). They urge that potential bypass patients be more fully informed, not only of the risks of surgery and chances of successful weight loss with this and other methods, but also of "the possibility that [they are] not behaviorally deviant, merely biologically different" (p. 470).

OTHER SURGICAL INTERVENTIONS

The lengths to which people will go to reduce their breadth is remarkable. Some people have attacked the problem directly, with lipectomy or surgical removal of fat. This procedure derived support from the now questionable notion that excessive fat cells *caused* obesity. In any case, patients undergoing lipectomy tend to regain the weight. Whether this outcome poses theoretical problems or not for the idea that fat cell number determines the level of weight regulation, it certainly does not solve any problems for the obese individual looking for a permanent solution (Bray, 1976).

Other theories locate our regulatory mechanisms in the brain, specifically in the hypothalamus. Cuts or lesions in the lateral nuclei of the hypothalamus in rats and other animals often cause virtual starvation, presumably because the animal loses its appetite or hunger, perhaps because its set point for weight regulation is lowered. In any case, none of the people who underwent lateral hypothalamic lesions exhibited any significant weight change after surgery (Bray, 1976).

Other approaches are limited only by the imaginations of the doctors who recommend them. These schemes—like lining the stomach with nonabsorptive material or having people swallow a balloon—are ingenious and appealing to those who have no reluctance to fool around with fundamental physiological processes central to one's well-being. As usual, though, the dangers far outweigh the possible gains. A recent scheme—jaw wiring, which prevents the dieter from eating solids—turns out to jeopardize one's teeth; one also risks suffocation if one becomes sick and vomits.

CONCLUSIONS

The direct adverse effects of the more dramatic types of dieting are by now reasonably well known. We have touched only on the highlights. The *indirect* adverse effects—principally, the fact that undereating tends to undermine one's ability subsequently to resume normal, natural eating and weight regulation —are less well known; indeed, we believe that we are the first to point out this hidden danger of dieting.

There are certainly many ambiguities in the research relating weight and eating to health. We believe that it is nonetheless fair to conclude that both overeating and undereating pose risks to health. Likewise, both overweight and underweight, in the actuarial sense, seem to be problematic. From an analytic perspective, however, we cannot confidently ascribe the problems apparently associated with actuarial underweight and overweight to body weight per se. Basically, there are two confounding factors: First, actuarial weights are complexly related to natural weights—people who are statistically overweight may be truly overweight (i.e., above their natural weight), at their natural weight, or even below it. When statistical overweight is blamed for a disorder, the blame might better be placed on one's maintaining a weight above or below one's natural level. The second factor has to do with the relation between statistical over/underweight and over/undereating. It appears to us that both overeating and undereating act as biological stressors. Many fat people and other dieters, even skinny ones, exhibit what we have called unregulated eating, in which the quantity and pattern of food intake bears little or no sensible relation to the natural regulatory signals of hunger and satiety. In the previous chapter we focused mainly on overeating; in this chapter, on undereating. As we will discuss in more detail later, over- and undereating seem to "cause" each other; and both pose direct health threats, aside from their disregulatory effects on behavior. Moreover, both seem to be inextricably tied to dieting.

BREAKING THE DIET HABIT

With the exception of the sort of weight loss techniques that we will detail in our concluding chapter, we believe that dieting (as it is currently understood and practiced in our culture) has very little to recommend it as a means to improved health. There is no denying that certain unhealthy conditions (such as hypertension or hyperlipidemia) are likely to be improved by weight loss; yet there is also reason to believe that it is the *absence of overeating* rather than the presence of undereating or the lower weight per se that makes dieting worthwhile. Eliminating overeating does not necessitate dieting, but rather can follow simply from eating in accordance with what one's body naturally requires. And, as we shall see, natural eating may prove easier to maintain than dieting, as well as healthier. The artificial caloric restrictions that provide the basis for virtually all diets—and remember, most all-you-can-eat diets are arranged so that one cannot eat all that much—seem to strain against the metabolic defenses that we considered in detail earlier. When one takes into account the additional problems imposed by the unbalanced character of so many diet regimens, and the specific dangers attendant upon specific nutritional deficits, one is forced to question the wisdom of jumping, almost literally, from the frying pan into the fire.

It is relatively easy to criticize the medical profession for its often thoughtless or ignorant advocacy of dieting as a solution to the "problem" of overweight. Some criticism undoubtedly has been earned. We are not convinced, however, that the proliferation of dangerous fad diets (or even dangerous allegedly sensible diets) is attributable to doctors' admonitions. The strenuous pursuit of thinness for the most part is *not* a reflection of how concerned dieters are about the morbidity statistics. As is well known, doctors' warnings are usually honored only when they accord with the patient's beliefs or desires. In the next chapter we shall confront the real reason for dieting, the reason that dieters may persist *despite* what dieting does to their health.

CHAPTER 5

Narcissus and Sisyphus — Social and Personal Aspects of Dieting

MEDICAL PRESSURES toward slimness, however prevalent they may be, are not especially effective on their own, except perhaps in those few patients who have experienced life-threatening medical crises. The fact remains, however, that dieting and the more general pursuit of slimness have reached epidemic proportions in our culture. If we discount medical pressure as the basis for most of the dieting we observe, we are left with one other plausible source: social pressure.

It is almost superfluous to document the extent to which individuals in our culture are exposed to insistent media messages, both direct and indirect, that slimness is a desirable state to achieve and maintain. Overweight characters on television and in films are for the most part either comical or villainous. Our heroes—and especially our heroines—are notably lean. Likewise, fashion models, who in a sense determine what we should look like—or at least what sort of physique we should have in order to make our wardrobes look suitably glamorous —are definitively slim. The January 1980 issue of the *Ladies Home Journal* quoted modeling agent Eileen Ford to the effect that aspiring models should be between 5'7" and 5'9 1/2" tall, long necked, leggy, and with an ideal weight of 116 pounds for a height of 5'8". The pressure on aspiring models to maintain a skeletal physique is legendary: fashion models are notorious for the nutritional abuse to which they subject their bodies. As difficult as it is for them, however, it is even more difficult for their public. Models, after all, are intended to set standards. When even the skinniest segment of the population has trouble adhering to the ideal, there is not much hope for the rest; yet the ideal, however, unrealistic it may be, remains in force, forcefully.

Lip service is periodically paid to the notion that diversity in physique is to be welcomed. *Vogue* magazine has editorialized against its own practice of using models whose slimness can only be described as grotesque. The editors have noted the increased incidence of anorexia nervosa in young women, and have implicitly accepted some responsibility for fostering unhealthy ideals. The "healthy" look that was promised as a replacement, however, has yet to make an appearance. Instead, the skeleton now holds a tennis racket.

One research team (Garner, Garfinkel, Schwartz, and Thompson, 1980) has examined the vital statistics of ideal figures with precision. A source of data was provided by *Play-*

boy centerfolds: over the period from 1959 to 1978, Playmates' body weights dropped from 91 percent of average (for age, height, and sex) to 84 percent. Similarly, Miss America contestants dropped from 88 percent of normal in the 1960s to 85 percent in the 1970s, and pageant winners tended to be even thinner than their fellow contestants, averaging 82.5 percent of normal in the 1970s. (These figures are actually in some sense overestimates, since the percentages were calculated relative to 1959 norms; since then, the population as a whole has become fatter, so that these "ideal" women are probably closer to 80 percent of average.) Thus, both the women that men ogle and the women that women ogle remain very slender; to the extent that some women may wish to be ogled, the message is obvious.

Examination of a related measure, the number of articles on dieting and losing weight published in six popular women's magazines during those same 20 years, indicates that these articles have proliferated as the ideal female shape has attenuated. The average number of diet articles per year increased by 73 percent over the 20 years, from 17.1 per year in the decade 1959–1968 to 29.6 in the decade 1969–1978. We thus have converging evidence that the ideal female shape has been changing to a thinner, less rounded physique; and, since young adult women have actually been growing somewhat heavier, there has been an increasing emphasis on dieting to lose weight and conform to the ideal. In addition to the standard "miracle" diets, the magazines feature countless mechanical devices designed to melt, pulverize, or otherwise dematerialize fat; for the wealthy, of course, there are the spas, where "experts" control one's eating and exercise so as to promote rapid weight loss. (One may also be entitled to a suntan at these spas, in exchange for the tuition; unfortunately, the suntan lasts only about as long as the weight loss.)

A final measure of media focus on dieting is the entrenchment of diet books on the national best-seller lists. The appearance of new "breakthrough" diets is scheduled, it seems, to ensure their orderly monopolization of the book buyer's dollar; just as one book fades—along with the weight loss it inspired—another comes along to take its place. More to the point, just when dieters are tempted to throw up their hands in disgust with the whole dieting enterprise, another wave of media enthusiasm washes over them, dragging them back into the depths of dietary despair.

Whenever one attempts to determine the extent to which the media pressures people into adopting certain values or concerns, it is legitimate to ask, conversely, about pressure on the media from its readership (or viewership). Most media executives are more than willing to justify their focus on certain issues, and their implicit or explicit promotion of certain ideals, as a *response* to public interest or demand. According to this argument, it's not so much that diet articles cause people to diet; rather, it's dieters that force magazines to publish such articles, through the natural workings of the marketplace. Likewise, movie stars *must* be slim, or people will not accept them as stars.

There is no easy way to determine whether it is mainly the media that exerts pressure on its customers or vice versa. In either case, it is clear that the social pressure toward slimness is pervasive. For any young person the least bit sensitive to the mores of the surrounding culture, such pressure will be difficult to resist.

Not many people do resist. As recently as the early 1960s, a nationwide poll in the United States found that almost a third of those who were overweight were not concerned about their condition. Forty percent were concerned, but not enough to do anything about it. Twenty percent were trying not to gain any more weight. Only 10 percent of overweight adults were actually dieting (Wyden, 1965). This relative nonchalance no longer prevails.

Not long after the nationwide poll was taken, a study of high school students found as many as 70 percent of the girls to be dissatisfied with their bodies and eager to lose weight (Hueneman et al., 1966). A few years later, another team of investigators found almost one-third of high school girls actually dieting on the day of the survey—even though only half of these dieters were overweight. A full 80 percent of the girls expressed a desire to lose weight. (Dwyer et al., 1967, 1969, 1970). In our own research on college students in the United States and Canada, at least half of the females qualify as chronic dieters; another study found that by 1977, 82 percent of college women were either on diets or consciously trying to control their eating in order to keep their weight down (Jakobovits et al., 1977). The young woman of today, then, does not need the media to inculcate diet consciousness; her peers will suffice. A nice example of the power of peer pressure is provided by an experiment that we conducted (Polivy et al., 1979). Female college students were placed in a laboratory situation in which we could surreptitiously observe how much they ate. Each subject was paired with a student who was actually an experimental confederate and whose behavior was prearranged. The results showed that when the confederate ate a lot, so did the actual subject; when the confederate "dieted," so did the subject. Even more remarkable was the finding that when the confederate indicated, verbally, that she was ordinarily a dieter, the subject ate less, irrespective of how much the confederate ate. This infectious diet consciousness, moreover, applied whether or not the subject herself was ordinarily a dieter. It appears that, in our society, at least for females, the mere mention of dieting is sufficient to trigger a self-conscious attempt to conform to the "ideal."

SEX DIFFERENCES

The reader will have noted that the dramatic survey results concerning the prevalence of dieting focus mainly on women. Indeed, there is little doubt that both the social pressure to diet and the responsiveness to such pressure is more pronounced for women and girls. No one that we know of has done the sort of historical and comparative analysis on *Playgirl* foldouts that Garner and colleagues provided for *Playboy* centerfolds. Still, one study of a wide variety of magazines found that men tend to be shown from the shoulders up, with an emphasis on the face, whereas women tend to be pictured full figure, with a corresponding emphasis on the entire body. This differential focus applied even in primarily news-oriented publications; indeed, it was even true of self-described feminist magazines. Another study (Silverstein and Kelly, 1982) comparing men's and women's magazines found five times as many articles on diet and body appearance in the latter as in the former. In the four men's magazines, there was a total of one advertisement for diet foods or weight loss products; in the four women's magazines, sixty-three.

As with females, there seems to be a close association between "media pressure" or lack thereof and men's responses. The same survey (Dwyer et al., 1967, 1969, 1970) that found 15 percent of high school females to be overweight and twice that many dieting, found 19 percent of males to be overweight but only one-third of them (6 percent) to be dieting. Compared with 80 percent of the girls, only 20 percent of the boys wanted to lose weight. Likewise, in our own research, we have found the prevalence of dieting (or concern about weight) to be considerably less in male college students than in females.

What is the basis of this marked sex difference in dietary concern? Perhaps women are simply more concerned with their appearance and especially with their figures: Certainly women's clothes are designed to exhibit the figure much more tellingly than are men's. The proposition that women are socialized to be more concerned about their appearance than are men is usually associated with the corollary that men are more concerned with status or achievement or some other dimension of worth; women, heretofore not allowed to seek achievement in more productive and meaningful ways, were taught to cultivate their appearance. Thus, the recent acceleration of the pursuit of thinness by women has been variously attributed to (a) their concern to avoid the "sex goddess" physique associated with the Marilyn Monroe type, enabling themselves to be taken seriously and distinguishing themselves from the sex-object standard; (b) an attempt, conscious or otherwise, to emulate a masculine (i.e., less curvy) physique, since women are now attaining success in traditionally male pursuits; (c) their concern to be perceived as being as attractive and sexy as possible (e.g., Orbach, 1978), but nowadays it is the thinner, less full-figured women who are considered to be most attractive. The fact that explanations like these are so widely offered by social commentators does not detract from their inconsistencies—for example, (a) almost directly contradicts (c), which clashes with (b)—suggesting that social analysis has not yet made significant headway in explaining the female pursuit of thinness. The women's movement is not internally consistent when it comes to issues of appearance, physique, and social power. Whether or not women *ought* to be concerned about their appearance, though, it is more than evident that they are. Certainly physical attractiveness is a widely sought after ideal, perhaps especially by women. And by current standards slimness is held to be an essential component of attractiveness.

PHYSIQUE AND PHYSICAL ATTRACTIVENESS

A 1978 article in the *Wall Street Journal* reported that in Tonga, a South Pacific island monarchy whose king holds the *Guinness Book of World Records'* designation as the world's heaviest monarch, men "seek the shape and density of a medicine ball," and women aspire to stout midriffs, enormous calf muscles, and enough firm fat to qualify as having "healthy fullness," the Tongan ideal. Needless to say, these ideals are not universal. Although we acknowledge, at least in our more broadminded moments, that definitions of what is attractive are somewhat arbitrary and vary across time and cultures, we nevertheless manage to react with remarkable disdain for body shapes that vary too much from our parochial preference.

Actual research on somatic preferences—which is to say, what sorts of figures, usually presented as silhouettes, are rated most (and least) desirable—contains a few surprises. For instance, most people believe that the reigning ideal for male figures is the muscular, large-chested, "Atlas" physique. In fact, women tend to choose a medium male physique as ideal (for, say, dating purposes), and very few are attracted to the muscleman physique (Beck, Ward-Hull, and McLear, 1976; Lavrakas,

1975). Moreover, there is some tendency for women to prefer men whose physiques are roughly similar to their own. Males —especially adolescent males—*are* more likely to choose the muscular male physique as ideal, but even among males there is a substantial proportion selecting the medium physique (Dwyer et al., 1969; Maier and Lavrakas, 1981). In any case, neither males nor females chose the thin masculine physique. Whether that is a cause or an effect of the lack of pressure on males to become thin is difficult to determine. In either event, one is forced by these data to distinguish clearly between pressure *against fatness* and pressure *toward thinness*. Our society clearly places more anti-fat pressure than pro-thin pressure on males.

For females, the situation is different. About 40 percent of high school girls tend to choose the very thinnest of the silhouetted female figures as ideal; the rest choose the next thinnest (Olmsted, 1981). Interestingly, the high school boys overwhelmingly preferred the second-most thinnest female physique, which suggests that at least some of the females' pursuit of extreme thinness is for reasons other than the attempt to appeal maximally to males' preferences. Similarly, college women chose a very thin female physique as ideal, whereas college men preferred a female physique a full size larger (Olmsted, 1981). In conclusion, neither males nor females prefer members of the opposite sex who are very skinny. This is not to say that *no one* likes the "stick figure" look in a date or mate—but such preferences are exceptional, as are preferences for a roly-poly partner. The average male figure and slightly thinner than average female figure predominate as opposite sex ideals.

Of course, even if it is not the very thinnest figures that are idealized, the ideals that do prevail provide plenty of motivation for dieting. Indeed, we believe that the pursuit of these culturally defined ideals of attractiveness is *the* reason for the dieting epidemic which concerns us. For most people, the presumed health benefits of dieting are just the gravy—low calorie gravy, to be sure.

But why pursue the slim ideal? Well, for one thing, the ideal is almost by definition what one strives for—or should strive for —but this is, of course, a circular argument, and it does not suggest why the ideal is so slim. We prefer to break the question into two parts, each one of which is slightly more—although not entirely—manageable: First, why do people pursue the ideal of physical attractiveness? And, second, why is it "thin" that is attractive?

One obvious answer to the first part of the question is that beauty is an absolute value, like truth or goodness, which doesn't require any further justification. But, although there may be some people who are simply interested in being beautiful—regardless of its consequences—these esthetes are undoubtedly a distinct minority. For most people, attractiveness is desirable because of something beyond beauty itself, either something that beauty signifies or something that beauty can be used for. Most of us are pragmatists.

What advantages does beauty confer? Well, as the very term "attractiveness" implies, attractive people tend to attract others. If positive social attention is valued, as it is for most of us, then physical attractiveness is of obvious instrumental value. One need not be a particularly penetrating social analyst to recognize that we become more concerned about our physical appearance when we are about to appear in public. Another clue is provided by the observation that the care we take in maximizing our physical attractiveness for others depends on who those others are, how well they know us, and what impression we care to make. The less well known we are, the more there is to be gained, usually, by ensuring that we appear attractive. The basic reason for this differential attention to appearance or attractiveness is that first impressions are necessarily largely a matter of physical appearance. The book, proverbially, is judged by its cover, both because it is usually the first thing we notice, and also because there is often not enough time to actually read a significant portion of the book. If we want to know what someone is like in terms of personality, character, and likely behavior patterns, and if we want some clue as to how we should behave toward that person, we must perforce make inferences from appearance. The situation rarely allows us the luxury of suspending judgment until such time as we can judge on the solid ground of prior experience. As we get to know people better, we become less dependent on their outward appearance as a guide to their personality, though we may become more adept at judging changes in their moods from alterations in their appearance. Many, if not most, of our social interactions, however, occur with people who do not know us all that well, or at least well enough to disregard our appearance in making judgments about us.

To be physically attractive, then, is to be prepared for social interactions in the sense of having an initial advantage. This conclusion, however, is both obvious—in that we all accept it as a fact of social life—and puzzling. It is puzzling because there is nothing *inherent* in a beautiful face or figure that should lead an otherwise ignorant observer to assume that the bearer of that face or figure is a particularly wonderful individual except in terms of face or figure per se. Why do we assume that an attractive figure implies an attractive personality?

The question why is still open to debate. There is little debate, however, about the general applicability of the beautiful cover–wonderful book principle. This principle has come to be known by research psychologists as the "what is beautiful is good" effect. A landmark study of this effect was published in 1972 by Karen Dion, Ellen Berscheid, and Elaine Walster. In this study, research subjects were asked to make personality judgments (e.g., assessing sociability on a numerically graded scale) about various "target" persons. These targets were completely unknown to the subjects; all the subjects had to go on were head-and-shoulder photographs of the targets. Unbeknownst to the subjects, however, the targets had been preselected, on the basis of the ratings provided by a separate sample of student subjects, to be high, low, or moderate in judged physical attractiveness. The results of the study clearly supported the "what is beautiful is good" principle: targets high in attractiveness scored more positively than average in personality judgments and estimates of future social and personal success; targets low in attractiveness were judged worse than average on these dimensions. Clearly, people are quite willing to make inferences on the basis of physical attractiveness, even when—or, perhaps, especially when—there is no evidence other than physical attractiveness on which to base the personality and social success diagnosis/prognosis. This effect is normally discussed by researchers as a "halo effect," in which one positive attribute (i.e., physical attractiveness) radiates outward and by implication subsumes various other positive attributes (e.g., friendliness, competence). Describing this halo effect, of course, does not exactly explain it. Explanations normally focus on the human drive for consistency in our perceptions and judgments, such that positive attributes on one dimension are assumed to go with positive attributes on other dimensions, or that people feel more comfortable when they do.

Whether one is born with a beautiful or ugly face, of course, has traditionally been regarded as a matter of fate—or parentage, which amounts to the same thing. It seems somehow unfair or undemocratic that people should be given such an advantage (or disadvantage) at birth. Still, as we are also aware, there is a certain amount of leeway in that we can enhance our own beauty; maybe people who work hard to achieve attractiveness should be rewarded for that achievement.

Yet it is clear that those who don't have to exert any effort to be beautiful also receive the rewards. This is true even in childhood, as Karen Dion has demonstrated: attractive children are likely to reap benefits not as readily available to their less fortunate playmates. Discipline, for instance, is meted out differentially. Less attractive children are more severely disciplined, and adults tend to have lower expectations, and make worse inferences, regarding their behavior. Indeed, the evident fact that beauty elicits more favorable treatment from childhood onward suggests that there may well be a kernel of truth in the stereotyped assumption that what is beautiful is good. After all, if our personalities are at least partially shaped by the quality of our social experiences and the treatment we receive at the hands of others, then it seems quite plausible that the positive personality assumed by others to underly an attractive exterior may well be brought about by the very treatment that the assumption encourages. The "what is beautiful is good" maxim becomes a self-fulfilling prophecy.

Whether or not attractive people really *are* better, because of the assumptions surrounding their upbringing or because of some actual direct connection between beauty of the spirit and beauty of the flesh, it is clearly advantageous to be physically attractive. The advantages are not unmitigated—for instance, beautiful people are sometimes assumed to be cold and scheming (Dermer and Thiel, 1975)—but they clearly outweigh the disadvantages. (Some social philosophers, such as Harry Belafonte—"If you want to be happy for the rest of your life, never make a pretty woman your wife"—may demur, but they are a distinct minority.) Indeed, people seem to benefit even from being associated with attractive people (Berscheid and Walster, 1974).

Most of the research on "what is beautiful is good" has focused on the face. However, parallel studies (e.g., Lerner, 1969a, 1969b; Staffieri, 1967; 1972) have confirmed that the phenomenon applies also to physique. In particular, fat physiques are severely derogated. Indeed, the current byword "such a pretty face" refers to the fact that not even a pretty face is capable of counteracting the negative stereotypic effects of obesity. The social derogation of obesity begins early in life and persists strongly throughout it. Even fat people tend to derogate others who are fat; they derogate even themselves, drawing stereotypic conclusions about what they themselves are like on the basis of their physical appearance (Millman, 1980; Orbach, 1978). Of all the possible physical attributes one might possess, overweight seems to rank among the worst.

But why? What is it about being fat that is so unattractive? It is difficult even for supposedly dispassionate critics such as ourselves to keep in mind that fat is, well, just fat. Fat is not inherently ugly. Yet, the association between obesity and unattractiveness is seemingly "hard wired" in our culture. What is the basis of such a strongly negative reaction? And why do we so favor slimness?

Unfortunately, our answers to these questions must be acknowledged as extremely tentative. Because the connection between physique and attractiveness seems to be so obvious, very little research has been undertaken to explore it. What research has been done tends to confirm the connection—but not explain it.

FAT AND THIN CHARACTERS

In the normal course of events, as we suggested above, we tend to draw inferences about personality from physical appearance. What permits this sort of diagnostic leap, of course, is our assumption that there is indeed a symbolic connection between our physical appearance and our essential nature. In the case of obesity/thinness, the assumption of a connection between physical appearance and personality is difficult to justify; on the other hand, there are some clues available to explain why it is made. First, as we hinted earlier, our personalities are at least to some extent shaped by others' reactions to us. Thus, if stereotypes exist with regard to the "obese personality," then it seems possible—indeed, likely—that some obese people will develop into the mold provided by the stereotypic template. We may be shaped, indirectly, by our shape. If the stereotypic portrait of the average fat person involves various negative attributes—say, sloppiness and gluttony—then the fat individual may play into that role. To the extent that stereotypes become self-fulfilling, the assumption that people possess various negative traits will thus develop some basis in reality.

Still, while the stereotypic "shaping" of personality may explain how a kernel of truth becomes implanted in the stereotype and how the stereotype becomes self-perpetuating, it does not explain the origin of the stereotype itself. What is it about fat that is so disreputable?

To answer this question, we must return to our consideration (in chapter 2) of the essential ambiguity at the heart of obesity. More specifically, we must consider the general public's confusion regarding the etiological role of behavior in the development of overweight. Basically, this analysis brings us back to the question of responsibility, guilt, and blame. After all, the public is well aware of the fact that one *can* change one's appearance, shape included. There is some societal awareness of the biological constraints on weight change; nonetheless, by and large the emphasis is on people's ability to change rather than on their inability. Thus, fat people are ultimately held accountable for their fat, both because they were somehow responsible for getting that way in the first place and because they are responsible for "deciding" to stay that way. Thin people, by contrast, are explicitly applauded for their achievement.

Our anorexic patients are perhaps the most pathetic victims of such societal reactions. Patient after patient reports that she was ridiculed or denigrated by family or peers for being fat (often when in reality she was at or slightly *below* a normal weight). Her weight loss, beginning as a "normal" diet, gets compliments and admiration from those around her. In many cases, the patient continues to receive such compliments long after her weight loss has become excessive and her appearance emaciated. One study of anorexia nervosa found that friends and relatives of anorexic patients often admire their skeletal physiques (Branch and Eruman, 1980), an admiration which contributes to the patients' refusal to recognize that they are too thin. One patient we saw aroused her doctor's concern when her weight went from 135 to 100 pounds. It was arranged that she would go to his office every week to be weighed, and call home from there to report her weight to her family. She, however, was determined to lose still more weight. When she went to the doctor's office, she put cans of food and other weighty materials in her pockets, a little more each week, so that the scale continued to register 100 pounds while her weight steadily dropped. Her family believed that she was fine and looked well. After some time, it became too difficult to hide enough weights in her clothing to maintain the 100-pound mark on the scale, so the patient stopped going to the doctor. For weeks, she would return home after her supposed appointment, and report to her parents that her weight was stable at 100 pounds. No one in her family noticed anything amiss until her weight had dropped to the dangerously low level of 75 pounds! Until that point, they were still admiring and complimenting her slim appearance. Social approval and acceptance of even extreme thinness, then, works in tandem with the devaluation of even minor degrees of overweight.

At the level of personality attributions, this emphasis on people's ability to reduce their weights breeds allegations regarding the presence or absence of that central, valuable trait—will power. Regardless of the fact that natural weights vary over a wide range, and that some people will regulate their weight at a much higher level than will others even while eating no more, fat is nevertheless assumed to be the visible token of gluttony combined with laziness. The public endorsement of this view might be difficult to appreciate, given the recent dissemination of research supporting the notion of natural weight variation (see especially Bennett and Gurin, 1982), were it not for the evident fact that people *can* change their weights. As we have seen, natural weight levels are not rigidly enforced. One can deviate from one's natural weight—and some people can deviate a great deal. Almost all people can deviate enough to convince an observer—including themselves—that weight change is possible. What is usually lost in the layman's analysis, though, is the important qualification created by regulatory defenses—namely, that increasing departures from natural weight run up against increasingly stiff defenses. What appears as an accumulating failure of will is in fact better interpreted as an accumulating defensive lessening of one's ability to alter one's weight. This is not to say that heroic acts of will cannot squeeze out a few more pounds of weight loss; rather, we simply argue that there is currently an insufficient public appreciation of the complex relation between the exertion of will, on the one hand, and weight change, on the other. At or near one's natural weight level, deliberate attempts to achieve significant change are likely to be effective; the farther one moves from the initial level, the less effective the deliberate efforts become. Because people usually start off near their natural weight levels, they are usually initially successful in weight change attempts—and they want to take credit for this success. Taking credit, though, means taking responsibility. The defensive limits that nature imposes on weight change mean that one should not take that responsibility lightly. The coin may readily flip from self-praise to self-blame.

Whether a fuller appreciation of the subtle balance of forces —behavioral and biological—involved in weight change and stability will eventually make people more circumspect in assigning credit or blame remains to be seen. For the present, we must appreciate the consequences of the current societal predilection to assign a disproportionate amount of the responsibility to behavior. From behavior, which we as persons control, it is a short step to personality per se. Fat people are blameworthy, weak-willed, guilt-ridden, untrustworthy, incompetent, and otherwise disgusting creatures (Lerner, 1969a, 1969b; Lerner and Gelbert, 1969; Staffieri, 1967, 1972). This constellation of attributes, of course, is not held together by a tight, logical thread. Rather, the attributes are related to one another indirectly, through their single common feature—a negative evaluation.

The societal pressure, the inference from weight to personality, the constellation of negative attributes are all evident in the comments made by a normal weight—and constantly dieting —friend:

> I feel like everyone is talking about me when I gain weight. I hate to go out and see people, especially the other girls at the office. I know how they judge everyone—if you're fat, you're weak and lazy, an object of pity and even scorn; if you're thin, though, then they're all envy and admiration. I can't stand the thought of everyone thinking that I must be depressed or in some kind of trouble whenever my weight creeps up on me. You may think I'm overreacting, but I know that they all notice if I gain a pound. Once when my weight was up a little I went bicycle riding (to get some exercise) and a guy yelled at me as I went by, "You'd better pedal faster than that, lazybones, if you want to get rid of that flab!" I was mortified. My whole day was ruined. I went right home and cried for hours. I knew he was right, though—I'm just weak and lazy. There's no excuse for me to have let myself go like that and gain 8 pounds.

No wonder people pursue thinness. First, the cultural emphasis on the behavioral achievability of weight loss makes such weight loss not only possible by definition, but mandatory, since anyone who fails to try to achieve "goodness" can be said to be "bad." Dieting is thus a cultural requirement.

Ironically, one point that seems to get lost in the frenzy to lose weight is the fact that the logical opposite of "fat" is not "thin"; it is "not fat." The disapprobation suffered by fat people can be almost entirely alleviated by their reaching and maintaining "normal" weights. Additional weight loss rarely adds much to one's presumed personality credentials. Still, the fervor with which obesity is castigated and the desperation with which weight loss is sought does not typically permit people to quit losing weight—or trying to—when the quitting is good. It's as if one found oneself with a fever of 103° and, in one's zeal to lower it, ended up trying to achieve a temperature of 95°. When all around you are engaged in the same pursuit, it becomes difficult to detect the folly. Indeed, if enough people manage to achieve body temperatures of 95°, it becomes difficult to argue against the socially *descriptive* proposition that 95° is "normal." In the case of body weight, of course, the situation is even more complicated, since we are arguing that the *prescriptively* normal level is not constant, as for temperature, but rather varies from person to person. This individual variation provides all the more reason to regard the universal pursuit of actuarial thinness with dismay. We cannot really endorse even "normal" actuarial body weight as a suitable objective for everyone (especially those with high natural weights).

To return to our original question of why thinness is so highly valued, one answer seems to be that fatness is regarded as unattractive, and so, by a process of logical inversion (and overextension), thinness comes to be regarded as highly attractive. But, as we have seen, the unattractiveness of fat is not inherent; after all, in Tonga fatness is admired. It is almost a cliche that thinness is the outward manifestation of inward virtue. But again consider Tonga. The defense of natural weight works both ways, as the Vermont prisoners discovered. Is not the King of Tonga thus to be congratulated for his dedication to the pursuit of fatness? Who among us can argue confidently that the king lacks any of the virtues we have come to associate with the skinniest of monarchs? It is only because in our society most people exhibit their feats of will in attempts to *lose* weight rather than to gain it that we associate thinness with virtue. This is not to suggest that fat people are to be honored for being fat. Our argument, remember, is that most fat people are either naturally fat—in which case they hardly deserve much personal credit—or unnaturally fat (i.e., above their natural weight) owing to disordered eating, despite or even because of their attempts to lose; the unnaturally fat neither expect nor deserve sterling character references on the basis of their "accomplishment." Still, one might imagine a naturally slender individual setting out to emulate his Tongan hero, and putting up with as much discomfort and discouragement as any dieter. He would be entitled, we believe, to equal praise.

SYMBOLIC ASPECTS

There is at least one sense in which the pursuits of thinness and fatness, in the face of regulatory defenses, are not symmetrical. As we suggested earlier, the defenses against weight gain may be less powerful than those against weight loss, for various reasons of evolutionary adaptation. Thus, weight loss, all things equal, may indeed represent a more "impressive" personal achievement. Another asymmetrical aspect, however, lies in the purely symbolic contrast of gluttony and asceticism. In personal biological terms, both of these traits may be unnatural, and not particularly praiseworthy. But, in the broader sociobiological sense, asceticism clearly provides more for the rest of the group, which may be a distinct social virtue, especially in times of relative scarcity. (One is reminded of the virtuous child who restrains his normal appetite when unexpected company arrives to share a now inadequate dinner.) The only time gluttony is likely to be socially virtuous is in diet groups, wherein the glutton sacrifices his own dietary ambition so that there will be less (and less temptation) for the others. The asceticism associated with slimness is, of course, largely illusory. Many slim people remain slim without any effort at all, and often despite rather large caloric intakes. (Likewise, many fat people stay that way despite the fact that they eat as little or less than their slim "heroes.") The fact that the symbolic values of thinness are in some broader sense illusory, however, does little to detract from the power of that illusory symbolism.

Fatness and thinness have myriad connotations, as social observers are fond of reminding us. For instance, it has been argued that the current dieting epidemic is in fact a reaction against the moral "permissiveness" now rampant in our culture. As indulgence waxes in some spheres of life (e.g., sexuality, consumerism), it is unconsciously countered by self-discipline in other spheres of life—and dieting is self-discipline par excellence. For the anorexic patient, as we shall see, dieting may be the only aspect of her life where she can enforce self-control.

On the other hand, slimness itself may be an indulgence. Some observers have remarked upon our growing societal concern with superficialities, with appearances, including personal appearance. A concern with one's own body, then, may represent more of a narcissistic self-indulgence than a responsible act of self-discipline. Again, the anorexic patient is often seen as avoiding responsibility by delaying the onset of adulthood; she refuses to grow up and symbolizes that refusal in the retention of a prepubertal body shape. Our entire society, in fact, has been diagnosed as youth oriented; and we might ask what aspects of youth are being celebrated. Vigor and freshness? Or self-centered irresponsibility?

Another important symbolic meaning of slimness is socio-economic success. In previous centuries, wealth was reflected by corpulence and the abundant serving and consumption of food. Only the wealthy and powerful could afford to eat enough to become overweight; thus, being overweight—or at least "well rounded"—was a status symbol. Now that food is more abundantly available and the cheapest foods are starchy, fattening ones, overweight has become prevalent in the lower classes. Now it is slimness that requires time, effort, and money to achieve. Not surprisingly, then, there is a strong association, especially for women, between slimness and higher social status (Goldblatt, Moore, and Stunkard, 1965). Since fatness is no longer an indication of a person's ability to provide for himself and his family, thinness has come to represent wealth and status.

These symbolic meanings can be listed almost endlessly. We still cling to the vestiges of the nineteenth-century assumption that slimness is romantic, ethereal. Also, forgetting for the moment about being consistent, we may note that slimness makes women more "masculine" and thus is of symbolic value to the woman trying to get ahead in a male-dominated world (Orbach, 1978). That slimness is presumably more attractive, and sexier, is inconsistent with this last interpretation; but it seems that symbolic interpretations do not have to be consistent with one another.

Why is slimness so attractive, so desirable? We have suggested many possible reasons, perhaps too many for the logical purist who might prefer one persuasive reason. At this point, we cannot really determine the answer conclusively. Different dieters may be motivated by different aspects of the allure of thinness. For many, there are probably complex blends of reasons. For most, the reasons are not all that well articulated, and possibly not all that conscious. Suffice it to say that the value of thinness, Tonga excepted, is rarely questioned; it is usually accepted as one of the self-evident truths of our world.

THINNESS AND SELF-ESTEEM

When people are asked their reasons for dieting, they rarely locate those reasons externally, in the surrounding culture or even in their immediate environment. Some dieters will acknowledge doctor's orders as the prime motivator, but the majority—which is to say, those who are controlled by social and peer pressures—will rarely if ever admit to the fact that their dieting is a matter of conformity to outside pressure. As far as they are concerned, dieting is *self*-initiated, by the dieter, for the dieter.

Dieters, if asked—and even if not asked—will generally identify their motive for dieting as a reflection of the simple fact that they "feel better" when they lose weight. This explanation suggests that the dieter would be just as diet conscious if alone on the proverbial desert island—and, quite possibly, this would indeed be the case. The connections between slimness and attractiveness, and between weight loss and virtue, are so widely accepted in our culture that people internalize them early in life and rarely have occasion to question them. Once they are internalized, of course, one need go no farther than one's own basic needs and motives to find ample reason for dieting.

BREAKING THE DIET HABIT

By and large, people do "feel better" when they are dieting —or, at least, feeling better is part of what they feel. Certainly, they feel virtuous, and expect others to regard them as virtuous: dieters are notorious for displaying abstinence in public even when they indulge in private. And, if the ratio of abstinence to indulgence is high enough to actually produce some weight loss, the dieter will feel better as a "natural" consequence of looking better. In short, dieting becomes a major component in the scaffolding underlying self-esteem. As one of our dieters put it: "When I gain weight, I can't face people. I withdraw into myself, become shy and unsure. When I lose the weight, though, I'm like a different person. I feel more sure of myself, able to relate to people more, to get out and do things." And it is not just social concerns that inhibit the overweight; they themselves engage in self-derogation. "People have the right to hate me and hate anyone who looks as fat as me. I . . . look at myself and say 'I hate you, you're loathsome!' " (Stunkard and Mendelson, 1967, p. 1296).

It is difficult to argue with feelings. In the last analysis, if the dieter feels better when dieting—whether because of feeling more attractive, more virtuous, more self-confident socially, or whatever—who are we to criticize? Whether or not there is a formal justification or rational basis for dieting—whether or not it makes sense—if it makes the dieter feel better, is that not justification enough?

As we have already made clear, we feel that it is *not* enough —and for the simple reason that dieters tend to get at least as much pain as pleasure out of dieting. This fact often goes unrecognized, though, as the dieter tends to attribute the pleasure to dieting itself and the pain to other sources (including not dieting well enough). We believe that dieting ought to be given its share of the blame; if this were done, then dieters might realize that dieting makes them feel better—and worse!

For one thing, as we have repeatedly emphasized, dieting is difficult—not necessarily at first, and for some people, not until considerable weight has been lost. But sooner or later—and all too often, sooner—the dieter encounters the tenacious defenses of natural weight. The good feelings of the early, easy period of weight loss are supplanted by the frustrations of fighting a losing battle. Dieters attribute the good feelings of the initial period to the wonders of dieting, the misery of grinding to a halt to their own inadequacies. As far as we are concerned, the truth of the matter requires taking less of the credit for success, and less of the blame for failure. Perhaps more to the point, the dieter should understand that diets by their very nature start fast and then slow to a standstill. Whether one then wants to regard dieting per se as making one feel better is one's own business; but it seems to us a very one-sided way of looking at things.

The inability to lose "enough" weight, then, is the first element in our reluctance to endorse the claim of dieters that dieting makes them feel better. The next element is the fact that actual weight loss is often not appreciated, or even accurately perceived, even by those most anxious to achieve it. Studies of dieters' self-images before and after weight loss (e.g., Glucksman and Hirsch, 1968) find that people in the "after" condition tend to overestimate their own body size, as if they cannot accept or get used to the fact that they are actually slimmer. More specifically, it tends to be people who have become fat early in life—people whom we have more reason to believe have a relatively high natural weight—who have the most trouble adapting, perceptually, to their own weight loss. One's self-image is not necessarily an easy thing to abandon, even if it is negative; one has, after all, developed a sense of self that incorporates not only one's values, motives, and personality traits, but also one's body. Giving up one's well-established body image may precipitate a loss of one's sense of self and result in some confusion. Indeed, it turns out that many dieters are surprised at how difficult it can be to have lost weight. One is forced to deal with a world wherein one is no longer fat— and all that being fat implies. Because physique has so many ramifications for social encounters, one must learn a new life. To some extent, this new life was the whole point of dieting, and should come as neither a surprise nor a disappointment. In fact, some of our overweight patients actually *avoid* weight loss because they are afraid of the "new life" a thinner body shape would foist onto them. One overweight woman didn't dare lose the extra 50 pounds that brought her into therapy because she was afraid that she would become promiscuous and ruin her marriage. She believed that her fat protected her from sexual advances by male coworkers and from her own desires in that sphere. Similarly, another woman was unable to lose any of her 245 pounds for fear that people would be able to get "too close" to her if she were thin. She saw her fat as a barrier and a defense against close relationships. Repeated demonstrations to such patients that their fat does not actually perform the functions they attribute to it, that they themselves do this, do not necessarily guarantee weight loss. The belief in the magical properties of thinness—whether they are desired or not—dies hard. However, "successful" dieters do learn that being thin does *not* guarantee social success, more friends, a better love life or career. If it helps, it does so only to the extent of not blocking one's path to these goals; it does not provide them.

Many dieters place all their eggs in the diet basket. If only they could lose 25 pounds, life would be marvelous. Diet advertisements to the contrary, losing those pounds rarely if ever solves the problems of one's life. When dieters begin to realize this, their reactions are often severely negative and inappropriate. They may simply despair, since dieting has let them down by failing to fulfill its implicit promise. Or, they may redouble their efforts, concluding that if losing 25 pounds didn't help, then perhaps losing 10 more will do the trick. Dieters can become somewhat crazy at this point, losing their perspective, forgetting their original purpose, and allowing their obsession with weight to overwhelm them, disorient them, and bury their true personal compass. Some analysts have explained the "neuroticism" of dieters as a response to their loss of their "comfort object"—food. Although that may have something to do with it, we believe that it is a more profound loss that bothers them—the loss of certainty that occurs when the instigating formula (thinness = happiness) is seen to be more false than true. In the long run, happiness seems unlikely to persist without self-acceptance; and, for the individual with a naturally high weight, self-acceptance and dieting may simply be incompatible. One might almost go so far as to assert that *any* dieting betrays some degree of neurosis, insofar as it demonstrates a lack of self-acceptance. Some (few) fat people, after all, appear to avoid the diet habit altogether; perhaps it is the neurotic conformity caused by lack of internal standards—a strong sense of self—that renders so many of us susceptible to the social and cultural pressures to diet. Maybe it is neuroticism that causes dieting—and the acceptance of some of its distorted premises—rather than the other way around.

This is not to say that dieting doesn't make things worse. As we suggested earlier and will demonstrate in subsequent chapters, dieting—by dissociating eating from normal hunger and satiety—breeds a form of artificial regulation that is highly susceptible to breakdowns and binges. Not everyone maintaining a weight above their natural level got there by dieting; some just never learned to use hunger and satiety signals properly in the first place. But if one is regulating one's weight sensibly, be it at a high, moderate, or low weight level, dieting (as it is currently understood) is almost certain to destroy that balance. In the next few chapters, we look at the consequences of dieting.

CHAPTER 6

Effects of Dieting on Eating

WHEN you feel nervous and anxious, do you lose your appetite or head right for the refrigerator? If you notice that it's after 12:00 noon, do you ask yourself if you're hungry for lunch or proceed immediately to the coffee shop? If you arrive at a party just after finishing your dinner and find that the hostess has spent time and money making scrumptious snacks do you say "No, thank you, I just finished eating," or "Well, maybe just a taste of each"? People who consistently choose the second alternative have what Stanley Schachter of Columbia University might call "the overweight personality." In a series of studies begun in the late 1960s, Dr. Schachter and his students and colleagues showed repeatedly that overweight Columbia students (and, later, Yale students) are less responsive or tuned in to internal cues of hunger and satiety than are normal weight students; perhaps in compensation, they are more responsive to external or environmental cues. In other words, the overweight students seemed more likely to act in response to what they saw than what they felt. If food was put in front of them, they ate, regardless of whether or not they were hungry. They also tended to eat as much as was put in front of them, stopping only when it was finished. Normal weight students, on the other hand, tended to eat only when they were actually hungry and to stop when they were full.

In one typically ingenious experiment, subjects were brought into the laboratory, and, since they had been asked to skip their lunch beforehand, the experimenters offered them sandwiches. Half the subjects were started off with only one sandwich on their plate; more sandwiches were available, the subjects were told, if they cared to get them from the nearby refrigerator. The remaining half of the subjects were given three sandwiches, instead of one. Now, if subjects ate on the basis of hunger and satiety cues, the number of sandwiches on their plates should make no difference; and, indeed, normal weight subjects ate roughly the same amount—just under two sandwiches, on average—regardless of how many they had had on their plate. In contrast, overweight subjects ate less than normal if they started with one sandwich, and more than normal if they started with three. These fat subjects clearly ate on the basis of the "calorically arbitrary" amount that they happened to find on their plate. They ignored their own internal regulatory signals.

Schachter calls the overweight personality "external" or "stimulus bound," since overweight people's eating seems to be controlled by the environment; normal weight people are "internal"—that is, they eat when their stomach says to. Furthermore, Schachter and his former student Judith Rodin carefully documented the surprising similarities between their overweight college student subjects and obese VMH rats. (These are rats with a brain lesion in the ventromedial hypothalamus —a lesion which typically produces tremendous overweight.) Like the overweight students, VMH rats are "external." They are more affected than are normal rats by such factors as the taste of their food—eating more than normals if it's good tasting and less if it tastes bad—its availability and the amount of effort needed to get it, and other environmental factors. Schachter thus speculated that both types of obese organisms have lost touch with their bodies and respond instead to the environment. Because of the similarities in insensitivity, it seemed likely that this external control of eating was caused, in humans as well as rats, by some sort of damage to the VMH. Since there was not much evidence to support the contention that fat people had detectably injured hypothalami, it was suggested that the structure was not damaged so much as functioning poorly despite being intact, perhaps because of some biochemical imbalance. In any case, this damage or malfunction was held to be responsible for obesity.

This is where things stood in 1972 when Richard Nisbett (another former student of Schachter's) published a daring paper taking these similarities and conclusions a step further. Nisbett pointed out that overweight humans and VMH rats are not the only ones who are "external." Another group showing this same pattern is organisms that are *starving*—that is, seriously hungry and/or underweight. Thus Nisbett proposed that what causes the apparent malfunction of the VMH in overweight humans is hunger or being underweight. Needless to say, the suggestion that overweight people are underweight (and correspondingly hungry) poses a bit of a problem for those of us who are accustomed to thinking only in actuarial terms. However, Nisbett argued forcefully that the actuarially over-weight might well be biologically underweight. In fact, he argued that this logical possibility was a practical probability, since actuarially overweight people are urged by society to diet. When they lose weight, Nisbett reasoned, they may fall below their body weight set point and thus enter, in effect, a state of semistarvation. The reason for the external responsiveness of most overweight subjects, Nisbett claimed, is actually that they are *underweight* biologically, not that they are overweight ac-tuarially.

At the time this theory was published, the medical and psychological communities responded identically to Nisbett's radical assertion—they ignored it. In fact, it seems that we were among the few people who read and were affected by Nisbett's paper. Not only did we believe that Nisbett was correct in his assumption that the so-called overweight external personality is really a consequence of the chronic hunger ex-perienced by overweight people trying to lose weight—and how many overweight people don't at least *try* to lose?—but we in turn took *his* notion a step further. If overweight people act in an external fashion because they have dieted themselves down below set point—which we've come to call natural weight, partially because we do not believe it to be a single point, but rather a range of naturally regulated weights—then what about people whose natural weights are not quite in the overweight range but who also diet, to achieve a lower normal weight or even less? Shouldn't these normal weight dieters also behave "externally"?

To test this notion, we developed a questionnaire which we call the Restraint Scale, given here as table 6.1. The question-naire is intended to identify people who, regardless of their

TABLE 6.1

Eating Habits Questionnaire

Name

The following questions refer to your *normal* eating pattern and weight fluctuations. Please answer accordingly.

Age_____   Sex_____
Height_____   Weight_____

1. How often are you dieting? (Circle one)
   Never   Rarely   Sometimes   Usually   Always
2. What is the maximum amount of weight (in pounds) you have ever lost within one month? (Circle one)
   0–4   5–9   10–14   15–19   20+
3. What is your maximum weight gain within a week? (Circle one)
   0–1   1.1–2   2.1–3   3.1–5   5.1+
4. In a typical week, how much does your weight fluctuate? (Circle one)
   0–1   1.1–2   2.1–3   3.1–5   5.1+
5. Would a weight fluctuation of 5 pounds affect the way you live your life? (Circle one)
   Not at all   Slightly   Moderately   Very much
6. Do you eat sensibly in front of others and splurge alone? (Circle one)
   Never   Rarely   Often   Always
7. Do you give too much time and thought to food? (Circle one)
   Never   Rarely   Often   Always
8. Do you have feelings of guilt after overeating? (Circle one)
   Never   Rarely   Often   Always
9. How conscious are you of what you're eating? (Circle one)
   Not at all   Slightly   Moderately   Extremely
10. What was your maximum weight ever?_____
11. How many pounds over your desired weight were you at your maximum weight? (Circle one)
    0–1   1–5   6–10   11–20   21+

actual weight, are dieters at least a good portion of the time. As you can see, the questionnaire measures two things—attitudes about eating and dieting, and actual weight fluctuations. (Weight fluctuations due to illness, pregnancy, and other non-dieting-related causes are not counted in a person's score if identified as such.) People who report themselves as often or usually dieting, who have lost weight in the past and have been some degree above their "ideal" weight, and who are concerned about eating and overeating we term restrained eaters, or dieters. Since the questions are directed toward a person's usual behavior, we assume that we are measuring a fairly stable, general set of personality characteristics rather than just fleeting concerns or temporary behavior. Indeed, we have given the scale to people repeatedly over periods of several months, and scores tend to be stable. Thus, our questionnaire is a measure that can be used to separate people roughly into those who are chronically attempting to lower their weight and those for whom this is not a concern. We assume that chronically restrained eaters are in fact fighting their bodies' natural weight. One can score anywhere from 0 to 35 on the scale, but we were initially reluctant to divide dieters from nondieters by simply picking a particular scale number as a cutoff point. Rather, we decided to be more cautious and to consider approximately half the people we surveyed as relatively restrained and the other half as relatively unrestrained. Over time it became more feasible to develop a simple cutoff score rather than looking at the distribution of scores in each study. Thus we now consider women scoring 16 or above and men scoring 12 or above—men characteristically diet less and show less concern in general about eating and weight than women—to be restrained eaters (dieters) and everyone scoring below those cutoff scores to be unrestrained (nondieters). This is what we mean in this and the following chapters when we refer to restrained and unrestrained eaters or subjects, and dieters and nondieters.

Once we had a way of identifying people who are likely to be below their natural weight—or, if not chronically below it, at least yo-yoing around it—we could investigate our hypothesis that the so-called overweight personality is not really limited to overweight people, but applies to anyone—regardless of actual weight—who diets, and who is consequently below natural weight or yo-yoing around it. Accordingly, we gave the Restraint Scale to a group of female college students and divided them into relatively restrained or unrestrained eaters. We then repeated an experiment that had been done in Schachter's laboratory comparing overweight and normal weight subjects. We, however, used *only* normal weight subjects, substituting dieters for overweight subjects and nondieters for Schachter's normal weight subjects. In the experiment, half the subjects in each group are made to feel anxious or afraid while the rest are not. Schachter showed that the anxious normal weight subjects seem to lose their appetites and eat substantially less than nonanxious normal weight subjects. This result is in keeping with the effect of anxiety on internal hunger cues, which are stilled by the short-term physiological effects of adrenalin. People who are responsive to such cues will adjust their eating accordingly—in this case, eating less. In contrast, Schachter found that anxious overweight subjects actually ate slightly more than did nonanxious overweight subjects, presumably because they were *not* responsive to the hunger-deadening physiological correlates of anxiety. (Schachter had no explanation for why fat people might eat *more* when anxious; he focused on the fact that they didn't eat less.)

In our own study, we found an analogous effect of anxiety on our normal weight restrained and unrestrained eaters. That is, anxious unrestrained eaters, like the anxious subjects in Schachter's so-called normal weight group, ate quite a bit less than their nonanxious counterparts. Restrained eaters, on the other hand, responded just like Schachter's overweight subjects; those who were anxious ate more than those who were not. Thus, identical-appearing normal weight subjects, differing only in restraint scores, acted in opposite manners. Whereas our nondieters behaved like Schachter's normal weight subjects, normal weight dieters exhibited the same behavior as had his overweight subjects. This experiment suggested to us that Nisbett's notion, and our own extension of it, was basically correct: the aberrant eating behavior of overweight subjects studied in the laboratory was probably not a function of their body weight per se. Instead, it seems that dieting is what causes the differences observed between overweight and normal weight subjects. As this reconceptualization predicts, normal weight subjects who were chronic dieters showed the same behavioral abnormality as had overweight subjects.

Clearly, this is a lot to conclude on the basis of one laboratory study. We did not stop with that single study, however. We have spent more than 8 years demonstrating that normal weight dieters respond to a variety of laboratory situations in the same manner as do overweight subjects. And, taking our analysis a step further, we too have done some studies using overweight subjects; but, in our studies, overweight subjects are divided into dieting and nondieting groups—which is difficult to do, of course, because only about 10 percent of truly overweight college students score as nondieters, so one really has to search in order to find enough nondieting overweight subjects to constitute an experimental group. It turns out, in any event, that only *dieting* overweight subjects show the so-called overweight (or external) behaviors. The few nondieting overweight subjects behave more like Schachter's normal weight subjects—or any other nondieters, for that matter—and tend not to show "obese personality" characteristics. We therefore feel confident in assuming that many, if not all, of the behavioral and psychological differences observed between overweight and normal weight subjects are actually caused by dieting, and not by obesity.

The remainder of this chapter will consist of research from our own and other laboratories documenting differences in behavior between dieters and nondieters. Although the comparison in some of the studies we describe was between overweight and normal weight subjects, bear in mind that overall our research shows that actual body weight is *not* relevant to the behavioral differences found. What appears more parsimoniously to account for "obesity" effects is one's weight *relative* to one's own natural weight—that is, whether or not one is fighting against one's set point.

Let us first examine the anomalies in eating behavior per se that chronic dieting seems to cause. One such anomaly seems to be that people who fight their natural weight do not respond normally to the full or empty state of their stomachs but, rather, eat on the basis of other cues. For example, Schachter and his coworkers found that overweight airline pilots flying from continent to continent were not bothered by the constant shifts in time zones, at least as far as their eating went. The normal weight pilot took several hours or even days to adjust to eating meals at the same time as people in the country in which he had just arrived; overweight pilots had much less trouble: they just reset their watches to local time and ate when the natives did. Schachter examined this clock-eating (as opposed to hunger-eating) in the laboratory. He rigged a trick clock to run fast, so that experimental subjects would think it was dinner time. The speeded-up clock caused overweight subjects to nibble more crackers than did overweight people with a slowed-down clock which said that dinner time was still a good half-hour away. (Normal weight subjects actually ate fewer crackers at "dinnertime," perhaps because they didn't wish to spoil their dinners.) Further evidence of this lack of hunger responsiveness was provided by a study which showed that overweight people had less trouble than did normal weight people fasting all day on religious holidays as long as they stayed in the house of worship. Once outside, in a world full of food cues from restaurants, bakeries, and their own kitchens, the overweight fasters had *more* difficulty maintaining their fasts. Presumably, then, for dieters, when food is out of sight it is out of mind. This interpretation fits nicely with the one sandwich–three sandwich study described earlier. In that study, normal weight subjects provided with only one sandwich were able, somehow, to keep the extra sandwiches in the refrigerator in mind, even though they were out of sight. Also, when they were given three sandwiches, they were able to forgo, on average, at least one of those sandwiches even when it was in sight. Fat subjects, by contrast, ate exactly what they saw—be it one sandwich or three—and, if they did not see a sandwich because it was "hidden" in the refrigerator, they did not eat it. To summarize, visual cues *controlled* the overweight eaters but not the normal weight eaters. And, to the extent that one's eating is controlled by one sort of factor (e.g., an external cue), it cannot be as responsive to other sorts of cues (e.g., hunger and satiety).

Taking this one step further, another experiment by Schachter compared how much people would eat on full versus empty stomachs. All subjects were asked not to eat for 5 hours

before coming to the laboratory. The experimenter gave half the overweight and half the normal weight subjects sandwiches and soft drinks to fill up on when they arrived, while the rest of the subjects remained deprived. All subjects were then given several bowls of crackers to sample and evaluate. They were required to eat only one of each type of cracker, though they were permitted to "taste" more of them if they wished. (In this type of research, eating is elicited in the context of "tasting" to minimize self-consciousness or other qualms about eating.) Normal weight subjects who were full, having just eaten sandwiches, ate very few crackers. Empty normal weight subjects naturally took the opportunity to eat a large number of crackers. Overweight subjects, on the other hand, ate a moderate number of crackers whether they had just eaten sandwiches or not. Again, their internal state had virtually no effect on how much they ate.

A final test of this "what you see is what you eat" tendency was done in our laboratory. Actually, it was done by one of our students who used a local French restaurant as the laboratory. Working as a waitress in a restaurant with a talented dessert chef, she classified her customers as overweight or normal weight on the basis of their appearance, with a corroborative judgment from the hostess, and then randomly assigned them to one of the experimental manipulations. Picture this situation. You have just finished a delicious French dinner. Your waitress now arrives and hands you and your party dessert menus. Perhaps you order a dessert, or perhaps you decide you have had enough rich food and settle for just coffee. (When simply given menus, most of our subjects, regardless of weight, skipped dessert.) Now imagine that when the waitress hands you the dessert menu she is holding a beautiful-looking piece of the chef's special cake of the day. Does this influence your decision about having dessert? What if, as she hands you the menus, the waitress tells you that her personal favorite dessert is the chef's delicious special apple custard tart? Now do you order dessert? And what if she is holding that piece of the chef's gateau St. Honoré while she urges you to try the apple custard tart? Do you still say, "No dessert for me, thank you. I'll just have coffee"? These were the four different "conditions" our subjects experienced.

Thus, since in a restaurant it is hard for food to be out of mind, we put it either more in sight, more in mind, or both, than is usual. Normal weight subjects, although they did order dessert more often in the last three conditions than when simply given menus, were far less affected by these manipulations than were overweight subjects. The overweight subjects ordered the displayed dessert much more often if they saw it in the waitress's hand or if she told them how good it was than when they simply read the dessert menu. It thus didn't seem to matter how we brought the dessert more to mind; once we had done so, overweight patrons were especially likely to respond by ordering that dessert, whereas normal weight subjects were less affected by what the waitress said or did.

All these studies show that for overweight people, their eyes are, if not bigger, at least more influential, than their stomachs. The reason this is true, we maintain, is that the overweight people studied in these experiments are so busy fighting against their natural weights that they no longer pay attention to the dictates of their hunger and satiety feelings. As we have repeatedly suggested, dieters *cannot* respond to these internal signals. For some, dieting requires that such signals be ignored; for others, dieting becomes necessary because they have been ignored all along. In either case, the control of eating resides not in natural physiological feedback, but in one's self-imposed,

calculated dietary rules of thumb or in the surrounding environment. As long as the dieter ignores hunger but exerts rigid control over what food cues are in sight and what is allowed into the mouth, this unnatural eating may seem to work. That is, the dieter may be able to ignore hunger, eat less than is needed by the body, and lose weight (at least until the body adjusts to the lower level of caloric input, as we described in chapter 2). Unfortunately, being out of touch with the body's messages of hunger and fullness may leave the dieter susceptible to other influences. In our society it is difficult to exert complete control over what foods we see or are sometimes compelled by others to eat. When these uncontrolled cues pile up, they may become overwhelming and the dieter's rigid control may break down, especially since this control is located completely in the mind, and not in the body.

We have done a series of studies to examine the effect of various situations that might interfere with the dieter's mental self-control. The first study involved bringing dieters and non-dieters to the laboratory for what they were told was a study of taste perceptions. College women who volunteered to be our subjects were asked as part of the study to consume zero, one, or two "tastes" before tasting and rating three flavors of ice cream. These "tastes"—or preloads, which is how we thought of them—consisted of chocolate and vanilla milkshakes. "One taste" subjects had to drink an entire chocolate milkshake, and "two taste" subjects had to drink an entire chocolate plus an entire vanilla milkshake. "Zero taste" subjects, of course, were given nothing. After this "pretaste" phase, all subjects were given three large bowls of ice cream (vanilla, chocolate, and strawberry). Their task was to taste each ice cream and rate it on a series of descriptive scales (for example, how sweet, or rich, or smooth it was). They were allowed to take as little or as much ice cream as they needed or wanted in order to complete all the ratings. They were left alone and given more than enough time (10 minutes) to do the ratings and eat quite a bit of "extra" ice cream. You may be able to predict better than we did what happened. It was our assumption that, as in previous experiments where subjects filled up before being given the test food, normal, nondieters would eat less if they had two milkshakes than if they had one or none, whereas dieters would eat a moderate amount of ice cream whether they had zero, one, or two milkshakes first. We were right about the nondieters, at least. Nondieters tended to regulate their eating according to their stomachs, eating more after smaller preloads. Dieters, though, responded to the situation just described in exactly the opposite manner from normal! That is, when given no milkshakes, they ate very little ice cream—maintaining their diets, presumably. But after one milkshake, and even after two, the dieters ate *twice* as much as they did after none. Every dieter that we later spoke to about these results immediately recognized this as what we have come to call the "what-the-hell effect." That is, the subjects had not simply been preloaded, as in previous studies using sandwiches; they had been forced to break their diets. Our subjects hadn't even fasted for 5 hours before the experiment, as had Schachter's; in fact, our subjects participated in this milkshake and ice cream study one or two hours after lunch or dinner. Thus, there was no way the milkshakes could be incorporated into their daily caloric limit. Once their diets were broken by the milkshakes, the dieters threw restraint to the wind and enjoyed their ice cream. (One normal weight dieting subject ate a pound of ice cream after two milkshakes!)

This study betrays, in a nutshell, the problem of dieting: As long as things go well, as long as there are no disruptions, one can keep the lid on one's food consumption without counting on the normal regulatory influences of hunger and satiety. But just disturb the system—disrupt the fragile mental controls, caloric quotas, and other gimmicks holding the diet together —and there is nothing short of one's physical capacity that can be relied upon as a brake. If satiety signals are not normally used as *the* inhibition of eating, their usefulness may atrophy; if one decides to use charted caloric quotas as one's guide instead, satiety cues may not be available as an emergency back-up.

Our first preload study had involved only normal weight subjects divided on the basis of the Restraint Scale into dieters and nondieters. To demonstrate that dieting status *regardless of weight* produced this "counterregulatory" eating pattern, we conducted a second study using overweight and normal weight college males. A special effort was made to find and recruit nondieting overweight subjects. (As indicated earlier, our surveys of potential overweight subjects indicate that at least 90 percent are dieters—which is why we're so convinced that the overweight subjects in the Schachter studies were predominantly dieters.) A small but sufficient number of overweight nondieters were found, and the milkshake and ice cream study was repeated. A minor change was that this time only zero or two milkshakes were given, as the one-milkshake condition didn't seem to add any information. Since both our normal weight and overweight groups consisted of half dieters and half nondieters, we assumed that weight per se would not predict how much ice cream would be eaten. This time our assumption was correct. The only factor that discriminated regulators (normal, compensatory eaters) from counterregulators (those who ate more after a *larger* preload) was dieting status: nondieters ate a lot of ice cream after no milkshake and little after two milkshakes, whereas dieters once again showed the (now expected) "what-the-hell effect," eating more after two milkshakes than after none.

Now that we were confident that this effect was a real one, we wanted to know more about how it works. If you are a dieter, you're probably more than familiar with the feeling "I've blown it. Why bother trying now? I might as well enjoy myself and start again tomorrow." In an attempt to show how these types of thoughts influence the dissolution of the dieter's normal self-control, we did another preload study. This time all the subjects were given two 8-ounce servings of chocolate pudding as their "pretaste." However, half of them were told that this pudding was a "rich, gourmet, pudding-type dessert," whereas the other half were told that they were eating a "dietetic, low calorie, pudding-type dessert." In fact, half the time the pudding actually was low calorie and half the time it was very high calorie, but whether the actual calories matched the description given to the subjects was a matter of chance—that is, the actual caloric value was independent of the reputed caloric value. The actual number of calories in the pudding turned out to have no effect on how much test food any of our subjects subsequently ate, whether they were dieters or not. However, what the subject *thought* about the caloric content of the puddings did make a difference. Nondieters ate slightly more after a pudding they thought was low calorie. Dieters, as we had by now come to expect, ate more after a pudding they thought was *high* calorie. Thus, just thinking that they had broken their diets caused our dieters to overeat, whereas thinking they had only eaten some low calorie, dietetic pudding allowed them to retain their control and eat very little.

We should mention that this study once again used only normal weight dieters and nondieters. However, a team of investigators in another laboratory repeated this experiment with both normal and overweight dieters and nondieters. Once again, dieting status determined behavior: these subjects, whatever their weight, behaved just like ours.

These later studies, in which subjects all received a preload but were given different information about its caloric value, should make it clear that dieters do not lose control after eating just anything: the preload must exceed their self-imposed caloric quota. In another recent study (Esses, Herman, and Polivy, 1982), we found that dieters ate less after a preload than after none at all. Presumably, this small preload was insufficiently large to render dietary success impossible; indeed, it seemed to make the dieters clamp down harder. When that small preload was doubled, however, dieters displayed their characteristic overeating, consuming more than twice as much as after the smaller preload. (The preloads, small or large, inhibited eating in nondieters, as common sense and our own previous data would lead us to expect.)

The evidence is pretty clear that dieters who are forced to overeat, or even simply to believe that they have overeaten, go on to overeat even more. The self-control, or restraint, that they normally exhibit is evidently removed by the idea that the day's dieting has been nullified. Are there any factors other than forced preloading, though, that might disinhibit the dieter's suppressed urge to eat? The word "disinhibit" brings to mind one of society's favorite chemical disinhibitors, alcohol. And, indeed, we found that whereas nondieters tend to eat less after two stiff drinks, perhaps because of alcohol's high caloric value, dieters seem to lose their eating inhibitions and overeat. (We have not done a similar experiment using marijuana but we would not be surprised to find that dieters are much more susceptible to the "munchies" than are nondieters!) Any disinhibitor, or perceived disinhibitor, then, may provoke overeating in dieters. Our patients' anecdotal reports bear this out. Alcohol and marijuana seem to provoke—or, for some, allow —the overeating that dieting presumably prohibits. Most dieters agree that parties—where alcohol and/or marijuana are likely to be consumed—are disastrous for their diets.

A separate series of experiments documents yet another kind of disinhibitor with which most dieters are probably all too familiar—emotional stress. Earlier in this chapter we mentioned a study in Schachter's laboratory which involved making overweight and normal weight subjects feel fearful or anxious and then observing how much they ate. As was mentioned, the natural response to this sort of stress is to lose one's appetite. Physiological responses prepare the body to deal with the threat, and among these changes are release of sugar into the blood stream, which not only gives one energy (to fight or flee, if necessary) but concomitantly reduces feelings of hunger. Recall that whereas Schachter's normal weight subjects responded naturally to the stress by eating much less than did calm subjects, his overweight subjects did not respond naturally.

The overweight subjects did eat differently when they were anxious—they ate about 20 percent *more* crackers than their calm counterparts. When this experiment was later repeated in a different laboratory the results were the same: normal weight subjects ate less when made anxious, and overweight subjects ate more. In this second experiment, the increased eating of the overweight subjects was clearer, perhaps because homemade chocolate chip cookies substituted for the crackers. We have also already mentioned a similar study from our own laboratory using normal weight dieters and nondieters. As you will recall, the nondieters behaved normally, eating less ice

cream in the anxiety condition, in contrast to the dieters, who ate more. It is interesting to note that in all three experiments, calm dieters ate *less* than did calm nondieters. In other words, when not made anxious or afraid, dieters stuck to their diets and ate less than normal. Making them anxious seemed to cause dieters to break their diets, disinhibiting their eating in a manner reminiscent of the effects of alcohol or "fattening" preloads.

A more graphic demonstration of the disinhibiting or diet-wrecking effect of emotional stress on dieters is provided by some observations we made in a psychiatric clinic. One of the commonly accepted symptoms of clinical depression is lack of appetite and weight loss. Indeed, loss of appetite is virtually part of the definition of depression. Yet we have frequently heard overeaters use depression as an explanation for their overeating. One possible resolution of this paradox stems from the fact that depression is alleged to dampen appetite because of its hormonal effects—which is to say, it acts as an internal satiety or antihunger cue. This is the sort of cue that normals (i.e., nondieters) should be naturally responsive to. As for our dieters, though, there is no more reason to expect them to respond naturally to these physiological cues than to any other internal signals. On the contrary, our intuition was that depressed dieters would, like our anxious subjects in the laboratory, be unable to maintain their diets in the face of emotional stress. Dieting requires that the dieter devote attention and energy to resisting temptations. Anxiety, depression, and other emotional pressures also make demands on a person's energy and distract one's attention from other pursuits. We expected that the emotional stress would overwhelm the concern of limiting food intake. Accordingly, we determined the dieting status of a group of depressed outpatients coming to the clinic for psychotherapy and asked if their eating had been noticeably affected by their depression. Depressed dieters reported that they were eating more than usual, and had gained an average of 6.33 pounds since becoming depressed. Depressed nondieters reported the reverse—they were eating less than normal and had lost an average of 5.33 pounds. The most parsimonious explanation of this difference is that emotional upheaval disrupts the self-control of dieters, causing them to eat and gain weight. Nondieters, for whom self-control around food is not an issue, react to the physiological effects caused by emotional stress by "losing their appetites." The moral of this story is that dieters should avoid tension and stress. Unfortunately, as we'll document in the next chapter, that's easier said than done, especially for dieters.

All the studies described thus far in this chapter document the dieter's basic failure to eat according to what his or her body is actually saying. Fighting the body disrupts other aspects of eating as well. In chapter 2 we mentioned a taste phenomenon (negative alliesthesia) being studied by Dr. Michel Cabanac and his colleagues in France. As you'll recall, they found that overweight subjects did not have the same declining response to sweet tastes as did normal weight subjects, but continued to rate these tastes as pleasant even after they had consumed a substantial amount of a sweet solution; the normals liked the sweet solutions only at first. The experimenters then tested themselves and found that they behaved like all the other normal weight subjects. However, they then forced themselves to lose 10 percent of their body weight, thus going below their set points, or natural weights. At this "subnormal" weight, the experimenters reacted to the sweet solutions in the same way as the overweight subjects had, that is, by failing to show a declining response to them.

Effects of Dieting on Eating

The phenomenon of negative alliesthesia was also investigated in patients suffering from anorexia nervosa. Dr. Paul Garfinkel and his colleagues conducted sweet preference tests on a group of anorexic patients before and after they had eaten. Like overweight subjects, these superdieters never showed the normal response of eventually rejecting the sweet solutions. Interestingly, when these patients were retested a year later, after most of them had regained much of the weight they had lost and were back at a normal weight (although not necessarily back up to their own natural weights), they still did not exhibit the normal declining response to the sweet solutions.

You may be asking yourself how important it is to prefer sweet tastes when hungry and reject them when not hungry. Why should it matter if people who fight their natural weight always like sweet tastes? A study by Richard Nisbett on overweight and normal weight college students suggests one problem. Subjects were given the opportunity to taste (and eat) ice cream. Some subjects got a delicious French vanilla ice cream. The overweight subjects in this condition ate substantially more ice cream than did the normal weight subjects. In another condition, the ice cream was adulterated with quinine, so that it tasted bitter. Normal weight subjects rejected this bad-tasting ice cream and ate a minimal amount while completing their taste ratings. Overweight subjects, although they ate more of this ice cream than did normal weight subjects, did not exceed the normals' consumption by anywhere near as much as when the ice cream was sweet and delicious.

Another study provided a yet more compelling demonstration of how the taste responsiveness of dieters may contribute to their eating problems. Philip Costanzo, Erik Woody, and their colleagues at Duke University used our Restraint Scale to identify dieters and nondieters. Subjects were given either two "high" or two "low" calorie milkshakes to drink, as in our earlier work—with one important difference. As preloads, half the subjects got normal milkshakes and half got bad-tasting (quinine-adulterated) milkshakes. Similarly, during the "taste-testing," half the subjects got good-tasting ice cream while half got bad-tasting ice cream. Nondieters, of course, ate very little ice cream after two milkshakes, regardless of whether the milkshakes and ice cream tasted good or bad (and, if they thought the milkshakes were low calorie, they ate only slight more). Dieters, however, overate the ice cream after they had consumed what they thought were high calorie milkshakes, but only when they had been offered good-tasting ice cream. In other words, even though the bad-tasting "high calorie" milkshakes made them break their diets—just like the good-tasting, high-calorie milkshakes—they didn't bother to go on and splurge after *either* milkshake if the available ice cream didn't taste good. Taste seems to be an important determinant of whether dieters will overeat or not.

In further investigations, we found another factor that influences how much dieters eat—the presence of other people. In all the studies on eating behavior that we've reviewed up to this point, subjects were always led to believe that no one knew how much they ate (except for the study we mentioned earlier where the effect of peer pressure was explicitly investigated). Every effort was made to ensure that the subjects believed their eating to be completely unobserved: food was always presented in quantities large enough so that it appeared that what the subject ate wouldn't be missed, subjects were always left alone to eat in a room with the door closed, and so on. These precautions were taken in order to prevent the subjects from feeling self-conscious about eating. Although we hadn't thought much about this at first, we came to realize that experimenters like ourselves clearly expected people's eating to be influenced by the presence of other people. Looked at from a different angle, all the things we (and the other investigators we've mentioned) had done to our subjects in these earlier studies seemed to have the general effect of making nondieters eat less and dieters eat more. The presence of another person, however, struck us as something that might have a different effect. It seemed likely to us that having someone else in the room watching them eat would make dieters eat less. Accordingly, our next study involved leaving the experimenter in the room with the subjects while they drank their small (5-ounce) or large (15-ounce) milkshake preload and then helped themselves to as much more as they needed to fill themselves up, which they were instructed to do. (Since word about our "tasting" experiments was spreading among the undergraduate population, we decided to have subjects "fill up" to give us a new, unobtrusive measure of eating.) We also had a group of dieters and nondieters who drank these small or large preloads under the usual conditions (i.e., alone), and they behaved as in previous studies. That is, nondieters took a lot more milkshake after a 5-ounce preload, and only a little more, if any, after a 15-ounce preload. Dieters, of course, did the reverse, taking more after they had already had 15 ounces than after only 5 ounces. When the experimenter stayed in the room, nondieters behaved exactly as they had when they were alone. Dieters, however, did behave differently than usual, although not in quite the way we expected. Instead of just taking a little more regardless of the size of the initial preload, the dieters actually behaved just like nondieters! With the experimenter watching them "fill up," they took only a little after a 15-ounce preload and a lot after a 5-ounce one—that is, they took the *normal* amount one would take if told to drink until full. Hence, the experimenter's presence in the room helped dieters to eat sensibly. However, this sudden switch to normal behavior lasted no longer than the experimenter's presence. After "filling themselves up," subjects were given bowls of nuts to taste (and, of course, to rate on various properties) and were left alone to do this. Nondieters, naturally, ate very few nuts, since they were full from the milkshakes. Dieters, though, reverted to their usual behavior, splurging on the nuts if they had previously had a lot of milkshake to drink, and eating very little if they had been in the one condition where they only had consumed a little milkshake (i.e., where they were not observed and began with a 5-ounce drink).

Clearly, the experimenter is a special kind of "other person" to have watching the subject eat. The sudden appearance of "normal" eating behavior in the dieters might well reflect a sort of obedience to an authority figure. Certainly, their behavior reverted to their usual splurge-or-starve syndrome as soon as the experimenter left the room. To see how a more usual type of "other person" would affect eating, we had dieters and nondieters (preloaded with milkshakes or not, as usual) do their taste ratings—and hence, eating—together with a peer. This is the study that we mentioned in the previous chapter in the context of peer pressures on eating and dieting. As you may recall, the peer was actually a student in our employ who played the role of second subject throughout the experiment. Under these conditions, dieters ate less than nondieters. All subjects, whether or not they were dieters, were very much influenced by the amount eaten by our "second subject," eating more when she ate more and less when she ate less. When she identified herself as a dieter, all subjects ate somewhat less, regardless of what the experimental confederate ate.

In a final study in this series, we found that the "other

person" didn't even have to be in the room with the subject. It was enough for subjects to know that someone could tell how much they ate. When it was apparent that the experimenter could see how much the subjects ate—because they were eating candies and we had provided no place to hide the wrappers —*and* the subjects themselves were being reminded of how much they were eating—by the growing pile of wrappers in front of them—dieters maintained their diets. Even after two milkshakes, they ate very few candies. Our conclusion from these experiments, then, is that dieters eat differently around other people than they do when they are alone. (Nondieters don't seem to be affected as much by the presence of other people, probably because they are not self-conscious about how much they eat.) Dieters are inhibited and eat a birdlike amount when they think someone else knows how much they're eating. They save their vulturelike overeating for when they are alone, or at least not being seen by strangers. The only exception to this seems to be when an authority figure—like the experimenter, or their mothers—stands over them and tells them to eat until they are full, in which case they eat a normal—neither bird- nor vulturelike—amount. As soon as the experimenter (or mother) is out of sight, though, the dieters "make up" for their normal eating by stuffing themselves with whatever good-tasting food is around.

What, then, do we know about the effects of dieting on eating behavior? All of the foregoing research can be summed up in some general conclusions. Most apparent and most important is the conclusion that people who attempt to escape the confines of their bodies' natural weight eat in an abnormal fashion. Instead of eating when they are hungry and abstaining when sated, dieters seem to eat for various cognitive or emotional reasons. Under most circumstances, dieters eat little;

thus, they are probably hungry much of the time, which may explain why they don't simply use hunger as a cue for when and how much to eat—they can't afford to. However, when they think it is mealtime, they eat, and they eat more if presented with a lot of food than if only a little is overtly provided; in other words, they eat according to what is put in front of them. Dieters eat a lot—one might say that they overeat—when they are emotionally stressed or upset, or when they have been forced somehow to break their diets, or believe that they have done so. Good-tasting food also seems to encourage these splurges. On the other hand, splurges are unlikely if only bad-tasting food is available or if there is someone else around to see how much the dieter is eating. If the other person present is also known to be on a diet, the dieter's eating seems further inhibited. If that other weight watcher overeats, though, it is likely that the dieter will join in and overeat, too.

In short, people trying to fight their natural weight no longer eat in response to the signals that their bodies give; instead, they are at the mercy of the world around them. Considering the superabundance of tempting food cues surrounding us and the social pressures to eat, often excessively, this susceptibility does not bode well for the dieter. Obviously, dieters can be more or less successful despite these factors. Some never give in and overeat, others do so only rarely, while some binge every day. Much research still remains to be done to find out why people differ this way. Are some people simply better able to fool Mother Nature, or can some dieters actually adapt to a lower weight, in effect lowering their natural weight more or less permanently? That is, if the weight one loses is kept off long enough, does the body stop trying to go back to its old weight? Will the abnormal eating patterns we've described in this chapter—and other side effects of dieting to be described in the next chapter—then disappear?

We do not yet have the answers to these questions. We do know, though, that if you diet much of the time and struggle to keep your weight below what is natural for your body, you are likely to eat like the dieters we described in this chapter. Going back to the questions we asked at the beginning of the chapter, we're willing to bet that if you are a dieter you tend to choose the second alternative in those and similar situations. Worse yet, once you feel you have overeaten or "blown" your diet, you go ahead and overeat even more. Your eating pattern, then, becomes a cycle of feasting and fasting in a merry-go-round that you never seem able to stop. We hope in future chapters to convince you to try getting off the merry-go-round and to provide you with a way of doing so.

CHAPTER 7

Correlates or Side Effects of Dieting

ALTHOUGH you may not have been aware of the various effects that dieting has on eating as detailed in chapter 6, you were probably not surprised to read about such effects. Having become familiar with the concept of natural weight and the mechanisms for maintaining it (chapter 2) as well as with the distinction between overweight and unregulated overeating (chapter 3), you may well have concluded that attempting to fight against natural weight should disrupt diverse aspects of a person's eating pattern. The "what-the-hell effect," the exaggerated preference for sweets and good-tasting foods, and the responsivity to the environment shown by dieters are all experiences you may have had yourself. Previously, you may not have connected these experiences directly with your dieting attempts, though. In this chapter, we will document some other side effects that you may not have connected with your dieting.

A survey of residents of midtown Manhattan several years ago indicated that overweight people report more emotional problems than do normal weight people. Laboratory studies by Schachter and his colleagues and from our own laboratory investigated this issue in more detail. Taken as a group, these studies indicate that dieters are more emotionally responsive than nondieters; that is, they overreact to emotion-producing situations and get more emotional or upset than normal.

For example, in chapter 6, we described studies done by Schachter and by us in which subjects were made to feel anxious. This was done by telling them that they would receive a very painful electric shock which would, however, do "no lasting damage." The subjects were asked if they had any history of a heart condition, and they had to remove all bracelets, rings, or watches from one hand. Furthermore, they were asked to make this their nondominant hand so that they would be able to write during the experiment. If this doesn't sound frightening enough, imagine how you would feel when the experimenter then attached electrodes to two of your fingers and turned a dial on a wicked-looking shock generating machine to its next-to-highest point. As we have indicated, this manipulation is very effective at making people fearful or anxious. All subjects exposed to it, dieters or not, reported feeling afraid. However, both Schachter's overweight subjects and our normal weight dieters reported even higher levels of fear than did the nondieting subjects. Subsequent experiments in both Schachter's and our own laboratory repeated this finding. It is thus clear that dieters get more fearful than nondieters in the same fearsome situation.

Another of Schachter's former students, Patricia Pliner, took this issue a step further. In an innovative experiment, she studied children at the doctor's office. Youngsters receiving their inoculations were rated as to how much they cried (negative emotionality) and how quickly they responded to the cuddles and comforting of an adult (positive emotionality). Inoculations are evidently very frightening for little children—overweight and normal weight alike, they cried heartily. However, the overweight children responded significantly faster to the comfort offered them than did the normal weight children. A second experiment by Pliner and her colleagues used a more traditional method to examine positive and negative emotional responses in college students. Overweight and normal weight male college students came to the laboratory and reported their emotional responses to a series of slides. Some of the pictures were simply neutral scenes, like a glacier, or a train pulling into a station. Interspersed with these neutral pictures, however, were two emotion-evoking ones, a nude Playboy bunny—which naturally elicited positive feelings—and an autopsy picture of a victim of a bloody car accident—which elicited feelings of disgust and anxiety. As you've probably guessed, the overweight subjects had stronger emotional responses to both of the emotional slides than did the normal weight subjects. When we repeated this study using normal weight dieters and nondieters, we found exactly the same results. A different study used tape recordings of upsetting descriptions of such traumas as the bombing of Hiroshima and how it would feel to die of leukemia. Again, dieters got more upset than did nondieters. Clearly, in various kinds of emotion-producing situations, dieters experience more emotion than do nondieters.

One of our studies offers some evidence that there are physiological concomitants of this excess emotion. A substance in the blood called free fatty acid (FFA) has long been known to be sensitive to stress; that is, when someone is under stress, be it from exercise or from watching a Hitchcock film, the amount of FFA in the blood stream increases. It has also long been known that overweight people have higher than normal free fatty acid levels. Putting these two well-known facts together, we concluded that the elevation of free fatty acids in over-weight people might well reflect the stress their bodies are under as a result of attempts to get below their natural weight. If this were true, the increased free fatty acids should be seen only in overweight dieters, and not in overweight nondieters; by the same token, the increase should also appear in normal weight dieters, but not, of course, in normal weight nondieters. When we analyzed blood samples from groups of underweight, normal weight, and overweight subjects, we found, as pre-dicted, that regardless of weight, it was only the dieters who had elevated free fatty acid levels. This suggests to us that dieters are actually in a constant state of stress, which may at least partially explain why they are so overemotional.

Such laboratory findings are supported by repeated clinical observations of tension or irritability in people attempting to diet. Nor is this the only evidence that dieting causes emotional stress. Since the early 1950s, psychiatrists have been familiar with what is known as the "dieting depression syndrome." It seems that for many people, losing weight triggers agitation, nervousness, anxiety, and sometimes clinical depression. These people are often distressed enough to have to seek psychiatric treatment for their depression. Some dieters on prolonged fasts have been observed to experience severe emotional fluctuations with episodes nearing psychotic proportions. Others report increased family, work, and personal problems while dieting.

Investigations have indicated that not everyone who loses

weight is equally susceptible to the sort of reaction described above. A few studies found no increases in emotionality and even found a decrease after weight loss was complete. The pattern emerges that people who become overweight as adults are generally much less likely to develop a dieting depression than are those who have been overweight since childhood. In other words, people who are probably above their natural weight when they begin dieting—those whose overweight developed later in life, probably in response to decreased exercise and slight but consistent overeating—do not get depressed when they lose weight. People who have always been overweight, since childhood—and whose natural weights, therefore, are probably those at which they *began* their diets—are the ones who tend to show the dieting depression syndrome upon losing weight; these are the people whose emotional symptoms—nature's agents—force them to abandon their diets and return to their original weights.

It seems, then, that if one is successful at fighting the body and getting below one's natural weight, the body fights back on more fronts than just the eating-related ones discussed earlier. And heightened emotionality is not the only weapon in the body's arsenal. Another, which is even less likely to be recognized as a side effect of dieting, is increased distractibility. You may have noticed that when you're dieting you can't seem to concentrate the way you usually do. Boisterous children or street noises seem to make it impossible for you to think or work properly. Several studies have demonstrated that this difficulty is directly related to dieting. A series of studies by Schachter and his colleagues examined the performance of overweight and normal weight subjects in response to various forms of distraction. In one of these, subjects were required to do a proofreading task while listening to various taped messages ranging from silence, to random numbers, to scenic descriptions, to emotionally charged descriptions of death and destruction. In the silent condition, overweight subjects actually performed better than did the normals. This advantage was reversed, however, when any of the tape recordings was played. Whatever form of distracting noise was used, the overweight subjects reacted by performing worse. (Interestingly, the normal weight subjects' performances actually improved.) In another study, subjects were made anxious—again through the anticipated shock treatment—before performing a variety of tasks. As before, low anxious overweight subjects actually outperformed the low anxious normal weight group on most tasks. And, as before, the opposite was true for high anxious subjects. We repeated these studies of Schachter's, using dieters and nondieters. Both anxiety and distraction interfered with the performance of the dieters, especially anxiety. The proofreading of high anxious dieters was atrocious. Nondieters actually improved their performance when exposed to either anxiety or distraction, and again anxiety had a greater (beneficial) effect than distraction. The evidence clearly indicates that dieting makes performance much more susceptible to distractions and other deleterious environmental influences.

Part of the reason for dieters' susceptibility to environmental interference may be that the thoughts and attention of dieters are more focused on the environment. Pliner performed a series of experiments demonstrating that overweight subjects do pay more attention to their surroundings than do normal weight subjects. One of Schachter's earlier studies showed that overweight subjects could remember more of the objects they had seen in a picture than could normal weight subjects. Pliner showed that this heightened attention applies also to sounds, although she also showed that the heightened attentiveness applies only to particularly salient sounds. However, these salient environmental stimuli can exert a very powerful effect on dieters. In one of Pliner's experiments she demonstrated that making a particular scene highly salient—by showing an object visually, rather than simply describing it—actually caused overweight subjects to spend more time than normal weight subjects thinking about it. The environment is thus more likely to influence the *thoughts* of a dieter. Furthermore, projecting the scene in front of dieters engaged their attention so strongly they actually took longer than nondieters to report pain when their hands were concurrently placed in ice water!

Another cognitive side effect of dieting may well be an increased preoccupation with food. Studies on starving people, including dieters, famine victims, anorexia nervosa patients, and subjects in starvation studies, have repeatedly shown that food deprivation is accompanied by an increasing focus on food in conversation, reading, thoughts, fantasies, and dreams. Starving men and anorexia nervosa patients share an interest in recipes and cookbooks, and a desire to become cooks or other types of food producers or providers. It is not surprising, then, that dieters so often complain that they can't stop thinking about tempting treats and forbidden foods.

Taken together, these studies and clinical observations of dieters' emotional and cognitive differences from nondieters present a rather compelling picture. The side effects of fighting against natural weight extend beyond simple changes in eating-related behaviors. Dieting also makes people hyperemotional, more distractible, and more tied to their environments. One possible mechanism for this, we feel, is that dieters are generally more aroused than normal. That is, the constant stress of trying to get below the body's natural weight causes the body to be more excited and agitated physically. One piece of supporting evidence for this thesis is the superior performance of dieters on proofreading and other fairly simple tasks when there are no distractions. It is generally known from years of psychological research on simple task performance that people do better when they are a *little bit* aroused, through interest, anxiety, or stimulants like caffeine, for example. If dieters were starting out slightly more aroused than were nondieters, we would expect exactly the performance patterns that were found. That is, on simple tasks, under calm, quiet conditions, the more aroused subjects (the dieters) should (and do) perform better than the less aroused subjects (the nondieters). However, anything that increases arousal, like distraction, anxiety, or increased task complexity—a variable that has not been widely explored in this context but which seems to affect dieters and nondieters the same way distraction does—should (and does) reverse this relation so that it is the less aroused nondieters who now perform better, while the more aroused dieters are too excited to concentrate well and thus perform worse.

Another indicant of elevated arousal in dieters is their higher level of free fatty acids. As we've mentioned, elevated free fatty acid levels are a physiological indication that the organism is experiencing stress; and stress, like anxiety or distraction, is arousing.

Even the heightened emotionality of the dieters may be evidence that they are overaroused. Increased emotionality is, of course, another side effect of overarousal, as anyone who drinks too much coffee (or watches Sanka commercials on TV) can testify. Thus, to a great extent, the side effects of dieting which we've described may well reflect the body's elevated arousal in response to the stress of dieting.

Elevated arousal, with all its concomitants, is not the body's only response to chronic dieting. As we have already discussed, the body attempts to reattain its natural weight. In addition to the metabolic adjustments outlined in chapter 2, and the alterations in eating detailed in chapters 3 and 6, we have discovered another set of reactions by the body to long-term dieting. These reactions concern certain neurological mechanisms called cephalic phase responses (CPRs). These CPRs are connected to the organism's response to food in a complex manner. Dr. Terry Powley has described in detail how these brain responses control hormones and other physiological reactions to the sight, smell, taste, and expectation of eating food. In a careful series of experiments on VMH-lesioned and normal rats, Powley showed that VMH rats have heightened CPRs in anticipation of eating. These CPRs control—and are thus measured by—the release of secretions like insulin and saliva. The heightened CPRs of the VMH rats result in increased insulin release, which in turn causes the organism to feel hungrier, and presumably eat more—though dieters, of course, don't necessarily respond this way to increased hunger. The excess insulin also serves another function in helping the body reattain its natural weight (or attain its new, deranged set point, in the case of the VMH rats). Insulin in the blood stream facilitates the production of fat from food. Having extra insulin causes the body to be more likely to turn whatever food is eaten—even small amounts—into fat.

We have attempted to extend Dr. Powley's work on rats to overweight and normal weight dieters and nondieters. We looked first at salivation, a CPR that is relatively easy to measure. Overweight and normal weight restrained and unrestrained college women participated in the studies. The first study was relatively simple. Subjects sat for 15 minutes with a dental suction tube in their mouths collecting their saliva. This gave us a baseline, that is, an idea of how much saliva is produced normally when no food is present. Then a platter of hot, freshly baked pizza was brought in and put in front of the subject for 15 minutes. The subject's task was to look at the pizza and periodically rate its attractiveness and their own hunger, while the suction tube collected the saliva they produced. The change in amount of saliva produced in this second stage constituted the subject's response to food, or cephalic phase response, which in turn indicates the body's preparatory measures for dealing with the food a person is about to ingest. Unrestrained subjects, whether normal weight or overweight, showed a small increase in salivation over baseline when the pizza was presented. Restrained subjects, again regardless of weight, produced about three times as much of an increase in saliva over their baseline. The dieters thus seem to be overresponding to the food stimulus by secreting larger than normal amounts of saliva.

Further studies have indicated that other digestive hormones and secretions show a similar pattern to saliva. Dieters sitting in front of attractive food show greater increases in their production of gastric secretions like motilin prior to and after eating than do their nondieting cohorts. Such secretions, along with saliva, are connected with the body's processing and utilization of food.

These last findings suggest that one of the body's reactions to tampering with natural weight is to alter its use of whatever food is ingested (even if it is less than the normal amount) in such a way that body weight will be maintained or even increased. Thus dieters who complain that they gain weight if they so much as look at rich desserts or take a deep breath in a bakery may not be exaggerating, or may be exaggerating only a little. As our studies on CPRs suggest, food is more likely to be used completely by dieters than is usually the case: if dieters eat *anything* after smelling or seeing attractive foods, they are more likely than usual to convert that food to fat. The thermostat for weight that we discussed in chapter 2 appears to be difficult to reset.

To this point, we have discussed the side effects of dieting —hyperemotionality, distractibility, overarousal, and so on—as if they were part of nature's revenge for one's attempt to tamper with natural weight. Another way of looking at the agitation and oversusceptibility to environmental stimuli, though, is as the dieter's reaction to the loss of internal standards. Dieters, we believe, are basically unsure of themselves. When it comes to eating, certainly, they can't trust themselves, in the sense of allowing their bodies to take over and regulate consumption. They must always be on the alert or their bodies will "make" them gain weight; it is no wonder that they are under stress. Moreover, the dieter who is unsuccessful—who has failed to significantly lower his or her weight below its natural level, but who has nevertheless "succeeded" in adopting an artificial eating style—is in equal peril. The problem for such dieters is not so much that they have defied nature by artificially lowering their weights, but that they have defied nature by adopting arbitrary, "external" criteria for eating. The fact that they may not have lost weight does not save them from the consequences of attempting to tamper. For they have entered an unnatural state, one in which they have become alienated from their own bodies.

The consequences of this alienation, as we saw earlier, are profound. If the dieter does not trust his or her body, the mistrust might in fact be mutual. Thus, the body, to protect itself, becomes anabolic (fat storage prone), even if the dieter has not lost a significant amount of weight. The threat posed to the body by a person eating arbitrarily and artificially is enough to trigger the anabolic defense.

As for emotionality and the rest, these may also be part of alienation. Dieters, after all, are unsure of themselves. They are struggling to reconcile who they are with who they are trying to be. Caught between these identities, dieters may well become nervous and overly dependent on external guides for action. The internal compass is untrustworthy; one cannot easily accept oneself. Indeed, one may have only the shakiest sense of who that self is.

CHAPTER 8

Results of Not Accepting Oneself— Compulsive Eating or Starving

As I left my mother's house I kept saying to myself, "I won't let her get to me. I'm not going to eat because of her. I'll just get on the subway and go home and wash my hair. I've had enough to eat today; I certainly don't need any more." But then I thought, "An ice cream cone would taste very nice and I really *deserve* to have one after putting up with Mother's complaints and insults all through dinner. After all, my brother won't visit her at all and I actually went and had a *meal* with her. I'll just have one ice cream cone and then go home." But the ice cream cone became a double scoop, and then I was off. I tried to stop myself but I knew I was bingeing and I had to finish it. I went to three different shops and had big gooey desserts at each one. Then I bought a half-dozen candy bars and some cookies. I was so embarrassed that I lied and said they were for my nieces and nephews, but I was sure the salesgirl knew I was going to eat them all. I ate them all on the way home and then collapsed in my apartment, sick and exhausted. I hated myself for giving in, but I couldn't stop it.

This is a description by one of our patients of what she calls "an eating binge." Compulsive eating binges like the one she describes are usually thought of as a problem encountered by some patients suffering from anorexia nervosa, who develop what is called the bulimic variant of anorexia nervosa. Such patients generally rid themselves of the unwanted food they ingest during their binges by vomiting, abusing laxatives and/or diuretics, exercising for hours, or starving for the next several days. But it is not only anorexic patients who develop this compulsive eating disorder, which is technically known as bulimia, bulimarexia, bulimia nervosa, or dietary chaos (Boskind-Lodahl, 1976; Garfinkel, Moldofsky, and Garner, 1980; Palmer, 1979; Russell, 1979). As the multitude of labels suggests, bulimia is becoming increasingly prevalent. Because many bulimics maintain a normal-appearing weight, they often escape medical/psychological attention. A recent advertisement in a London newspaper seeking bulimics attracted over a thousand responses, while in Chicago an article about bulimia and a local treatment center for it drew thousands of letters from bulimics requesting information or treatment. Most of these people were women, very few had ever been treated for their problem, and many had been gorging and purging as often as six times a day for as long as 10 years or more! Bulimia seems to be a widespread and serious problem.

Furthermore, bulimia does not appear to occur randomly. Bingers tend overwhelmingly to be female and generally range in age from the teens to the thirties. This corresponds to the segment of the population in which dieting is most prevalent, and, indeed, most binge eaters seem also to be dieters. We do not consider this correspondence to be coincidental, nor do we believe, as most people seem to, that binge eaters are dieters because they have to diet in order to compensate for their overeating. The logic of our times would seem to argue that dieting follows overeating as inexorably as Monday follows the weekend. We have argued for some time (Polivy, Herman, Olmsted, and Jazwinski, 1982), however, that dieting is the cause, rather than the effect, of binge eating. Insofar as this "obvious" relation has been scientifically investigated, the evidence supports the thesis that dieting precedes binge eating, rather than following it. As we mentioned above, self-starving anorexia nervosa patients often develop binge eating, apparently as part of their anorexic syndrome. In fact, approximately 50 percent of anorexia nervosa patients seem to become binge eaters (Garfinkel, Moldofsky, and Garner, 1980). Cases where it is possible to reconstruct the temporal sequence of symptom development show that the dieting precedes the binge eating, often by many months (Casper et al., 1980; Garfinkel et al., 1980; Russell, 1979). Binge eaters who have not had anorexia nervosa also report that their binge eating began after a period of dieting (Boskind-Lodahl, 1976; Pyle, Mitchell, and Eckert, 1981). Similarly, formerly overweight people who have dieted successfully and become thin often report that they "either diet or go hog wild on sweets and all that stuff" (Bruch, 1973, p. 200). Such clinical observations of people who have actually sought help for their binge eating clearly suggest that dieting comes before, and probably produces, binge eating.

Experimental studies where people are induced to diet or lose weight are rare, but one outstanding example—the Minnesota conscientious objector starvation study—has been discussed in previous chapters. This study supports our hypothesis perfectly (see, e.g., Franklin et al., 1948). The normal young men who participated in this study had certainly not previously been either dieters or binge eaters. After starving themselves down to approximately 74 percent of their normal weight, these men were refed and returned to their prior normal levels. *After* reaching their normal weight, however, the conscientious objectors began to gorge themselves, eating as much food as they could hold at mealtimes, despite the now unlimited availability of food. As the investigators observed, "attempts to avoid wasting even a particle [of food] continued in the face of unlimited supplies of immediately available food. An irrational fear that food would somehow be taken away from them was present in some of the men. This may have motivated their [observed behavior of] eating as much as they could hold at any given time" (Franklin et al., 1948, p. 38). Thus, even when they were no longer deprived, dieting, or underweight, the men "ate more food than they were prepared to cope with," making themselves actually ill—just like the typical binge eaters. And, in this case, there is no gainsaying that the dieting led to the overeating; there was no other plausible cause.

Viewed in this context, the experiments reported earlier on overeating in restrained eaters take on a new meaning. The counterregulation, or overeating, of supposedly normal dieting college students appears to reflect this proclivity of dieters toward binge eating. When forced to overeat or break their diets, or when in any other disinhibitory situation, dieters out-eat both their nondieting counterparts and other, unmolested, nondisinhibited dieters. If such overeating is even manifested in a place as unnatural and public as a laboratory, how much stronger might the effect be in the privacy of one's real life?

It thus seems that dieting—even nonpathological, "normal" dieting, as practiced by at least half the female college students in the country—produces compulsive overeating, which in many cases reaches the proportions of true clinical binge eating. This, then, is another virtually unrecognized danger attached to dieting. For a large number of people, the voluntary restrictions of dieting trigger what becomes an involuntary, uncontrolled cycle of dieting and gorging.

Compulsive eating is mirrored by the opposite extreme, compulsive refusal to eat, the most widely recognized characteristic of anorexia nervosa. One of our patients describes her struggle to eat as follows:

I sat down at the kitchen table with a peanut butter sandwich. I had bought the peanut butter myself at the health food store so I thought I would feel okay about eating it. I can't bring myself to eat food anyone else has bought or prepared. It makes me feel like gagging or choking. But this was my own food, I paid for it myself. I took a bite and chewed it very slowly. Then I swallowed it, and I felt like it might be all right. After a few more bites, though, my stomach felt bloated and full and I could feel those three bites of bread and peanut butter inside me. My stomach began to feel all twisted, like it was tied in knots, and I couldn't force down another bite. I know that's not enough to make me gain any weight, but I started feeling fat. I realized I wasn't worthy of food, I didn't deserve to eat. I tried to take another bite but I couldn't do it. I stared and stared at that sandwich until I started to cry. I felt humiliated, defeated—I promised to gain a pound this week but I knew I could never do it. I had failed again.

Initially, when they are losing weight, anorexic patients tend to feel exhilarated, powerful, and triumphant. As another of our patients put it, "My mother said that if I wouldn't eat, she wouldn't eat. She said if I insisted on starving I would be making her starve too. But I still wouldn't eat, because I knew she couldn't do it. And I was right! By the next morning she had broken down and eaten. I was eating less and less, but I felt stronger and stronger. I was in control!" But this feeling tends not to last. As the initial compliments on her slimness become complaints that she is too thin and pleas or demands that she eat more, the anorexic tends to feel more and more driven. Although the scale maintains that she is still losing weight and is skinny, she becomes even more convinced that she is fat. After prolonged struggles (often over years), some anorexics reach the point described by our first anorexic patient. They finally accept that they are too thin but are still unable to force themselves to eat and gain weight.

For both the anorexics and the bulimics, the possibility of choice seems out of reach. They often don't want—at least consciously—to continue their self-destructive eating patterns, and they feel humiliated and defeated by their inability to control themselves, to eat "normally." But they are compelled; they are compulsive eaters or noneaters. Eating and hunger have somehow become dissociated for these people. Bulimics binge whether they are hungry or sated, and often they are sated and they know it. Anorexics view hunger as a sign that they are losing weight and often enjoy it. For both groups, eating becomes a symbolic activity of sorts. For anorexics, eating may represent weakness, giving in, or lack of control, or it may represent a normalcy they somehow don't deserve. Their inability to eat is both a triumph and a curse; it represents their dramatically heightened self-control, while at the same time it is beyond their control. Compulsive binge eating may also be a form of self-punishment, or it may represent all the "treats" which have been unavailable or denied in other spheres, a gorging on goodies that were deserved but had never been received. In either case, food becomes the focus of life—eating and avoiding eating dominate the person's waking hours. As a bulimic anorexia nervosa patient observed,

> My whole life centers on food. If I'm bingeing, all my time is spent getting food, eating it, and then trying to get rid of it and worrying about whether I got it all or will get fat. If I'm starving, I'm constantly thinking about food, trying to decide when to eat so as not to be hungry, but making sure not to eat too early so I'll last until my next meal, and trying to figure out what to eat that will satisfy me without making me feel guilty and trigger another binge. Even if I'm doing really well [i.e., starving, not eating at all] and feel light and empty, I can't seem to get rid of food thoughts. I find myself thinking about tasty meals or a particular treat, and I can't seem to concentrate on anything else. Whether I'm eating or not, bingeing or starving, all I can think about is food!

Such obsessions with food and eating seem to characterize starving people in general (even dieters or self-starvers). Underfed concentration camp inmates reportedly talked and fantasized frequently about meals and foods now inaccessible to them. Similarly, the Minnesota conscientious objectors in their starved state not only talked about food, but began collecting recipes; some even decided to become chefs after the experiment (Franklin et al., 1948). Emaciated anorexia nervosa patients also collect recipes; they become gourmet cooks—forcing *others* to eat their prodigious, mouthwatering meals—or choose food-related careers, preparing or serving to others what they themselves are unwilling or unable to eat (Bruch, 1978).

Such ruminating about food is often accompanied by what

is called dichotomous thinking (Garfinkel and Garner, 1982), identified originally in anorexia nervosa patients. Dichotomous thinking involves the perception of foods as either "good," diet foods or "bad," fattening foods; there are "good," small, low calorie amounts or large, diet-breaking, "binge" amounts. Such black-or-white thinking probably contributes to the starve-or-binge pattern of eating described in chapter 6 as characteristic of dieters. Under normal circumstances, dieters eat less than nondieters; that is, they eat small, "diet" amounts of food. Under any kind of disinhibition, however, be it anxiety, depression, alcohol, or the belief that one has already transgressed the diet's boundaries (i.e., eaten "bad" food or "bad" amounts), dieters overeat or even binge. The mere belief, true or not, that one has "broken the diet" is sufficient to trigger overeating in someone who thinks only in terms of diet versus binge.

Bingers come in all shapes and sizes—thin, normal, and obese. Similarly, many anorexics eat their way out of the hospital and even into obesity without resolving the problems that initiated their anorexia nervosa; so anorexics ultimately come in all shapes and sizes as well. It thus becomes rather simplistic to argue that excessive thinness or fatness is caused by any single factor, such as avoiding sexuality or cultivating it. (Both arguments have been made at various times for both extremes of body size.) Other single-focused "causes" for the problems are equally if not more unsophisticated. Eating disorders (in either direction) seem to be multidetermined rather than having unitary causes (Garfinkel and Garner, 1982); some of these causes may be unique to a particular problem whereas others are shared. What eating problems in both directions do have in common is the compulsive, driven, out-of-control nature of the behaviors involved, and the underlying attempt to solve one's problems or change oneself through eating, weight loss, or weight gain.

So, while any particular eating disorder has a variety of different causes or predisposing factors in different victims, some commonalities emerge across both individuals and problems. Anorexia nervosa, compulsive or binge eating, and obesity all seem to share a similar, underlying misperception that food, eating, and/or body shape can solve any kind of problem and improve one's life. This is clearly a mistaken belief, since even changing one's weight does not change one's identity. Rarely, if ever, is weight change the actual factor that results in an improved existence—despite the fact that people may ascribe changes in their life circumstances to changes in their weights. Moreover, food never solves problems unrelated to hunger. At best, it sedates one, like a drug, or distracts the mind temporarily; at worst, it adds new problems, like overweight, guilt, or a need for money to buy more food. Nevertheless, countless people attempt to use food and eating for purposes other than physical nourishment.

Over 25 years ago, the psychosomatic theory of obesity posited that obesity results from overeating initiated by psychic or emotional states rather than hunger (Hamburger, 1951; Kaplan and Kaplan, 1957). In other words, excessive food intake is instigated by appetite—the psychological desire to eat— rather than by hunger—the physiological sensations reflecting the body's need for food (Hamburger, 1951). Commonly, emotional states affect both appetite and hunger; many people find themselves unable to eat when they are angry, depressed, afraid, or otherwise upset. Physiological responses to these emotional states often include the release of stored sugar into the blood stream, which generally reduces hunger. The reason appetite tends to diminish is perhaps that the emotion is too riveting to allow such mundane matters as food to intrude (as the person falling in love will attest). However, as we have seen, for some people these emotional states seem to foster an *increased* appetite. Overweight people have repeatedly been found to overeat when they are upset (Bruch, 1957; Hamburger, 1951; Kaplan and Kaplan, 1957). Clinical evidence suggests that some people—overweight or otherwise—overeat as a response to emotional tensions or upsets (Bruch, 1957; Hamburger, 1951; Kaplan and Kaplan, 1957), as a form of gratification during frustrating or intolerable life events (Bruch, 1957; Kaplan and Kaplan, 1957), as a kind of sedative or tranquilizer (Brosin, 1954; Feinstein, 1960, Glucksman and Hirsch, 1968), as a symptom of depression or depressive equivalent (Bruch, 1957; Simon, 1963), or as a chronic substitute for some ungratified need such as the need for love or affection (Bruch, 1957; Orbach, 1978).

Even people who manage to lose weight become more likely to regain it if they are prone to snacking in situations where they are emotionally aroused but not actually hungry (Leon and Chamberlain, 1973a, 1973b). Our own work similarly suggests that emotionally triggered overeating is not limited to the overweight. Recall, for example, the study in which we asked a group of depressed patients at a psychiatric clinic whether they had lost or gained weight since their depression began; we found that unrestrained, nondieter depressed patients had lost weight, while the restrained, dieter depressives had gained weight (Polivy and Herman, 1976). Later work supports this finding that it is degree of dietary restraint, not degree of overweight, which predicts who gains weight when depressed (Zielinsky, 1978).

Similarly, numerous laboratory studies have demonstrated that, in contrast to unrestrained college students, overweight and normal weight restrained students do not decrease their eating when made anxious or depressed (Abramson and Wunderlich, 1972; Schachter, Goldman, and Gordon, 1968); in fact, they often overeat in such circumstances (Ely et al., 1979; Herman and Polivy, 1975; McKenna, 1972; Slochower, 1976). In all such studies, the anxious/depressed overweight or dieting subjects ate more than their nondieting counterparts. Thus, both the clinical and laboratory studies indicate that overweight people and dieters—or as we would argue, dieters regardless of their weight—are more prone than are nondieters to eat in emotional situations, or for reasons other than hunger.

It has been argued that this inappropriate eating reflects a lack of responsiveness to internal bodily signals of hunger or satiety, and that these people may either lack or be unaware of such signals (Schachter and Rodin, 1974). Or, it may be as our work in chapter 6 suggests, that the signals are present to a normal degree but are ignored because they interfere with attempted dieting (by making the person "hungrier" than carrot and celery sticks can satisfy; see Polivy, Herman, and Warsh, 1978). If one is trying to reduce to below natural weight, normal hunger signals would call for an amount of food intake that would prevent this weight loss. It would thus be necessary to ignore one's hunger signals in order to eat sufficiently little for weight loss to occur. As the body tends to adjust to the decreased food supply by becoming more efficient in its use of what food is available (as we discussed in chapter 2), the dieter must take in even less food to keep losing weight. Normal hunger signals would then become even more treacherous to the unwary dieter, and so it is increasingly advantageous to ignore such signals entirely. Dieting thus virtually requires a lack of responsiveness to internal hunger cues, thereby severing the usual relation between hunger and eating.

In this way, eating for reasons other than hunger becomes a distinct possibility, since satiety signals would tend to be ignored along with hunger signals. The overeating that occurs when the diet is broken may well reflect this process of detachment from internal hunger and satiety signals.

There are other types of eating not really instigated by hunger which may reflect a completely different process. The emotion-induced eating we have just discussed may reflect a *confusion* between the internal signals of hunger and the internal signals of emotion, with emotional signals "taking over" from hunger signals, as has been theorized (Bruch, 1973). If emotional distress were met, from infancy on, by an offer of food —"Don't cry, baby; here's a cookie. Now don't you feel better?" or "The baby's crying; I'd better feed it"—then the person may have simply learned an association between food and emotion, or may confuse the feelings of emotion with those of hunger, since emotion always meant that one ate, just as hunger did. Alternatively, if food were always offered as a sedative to soothe distress, the person may continue to calm down with a cookie—or a box of cookies. Even good feelings may trigger such inappropriate eating if food has been used as a reward in childhood—"If you're good, you can have ice cream." Thus, early training may contribute to inappropriate eating in adulthood. Long association of food and emotional states can lead to a confusion of hunger and emotionality—a sense that emotional states somehow call for food, even though the person does recognize the distinction between emotion and actual hunger—or to the misuse of food as a sedative or reward. In the passages quoted earlier in this chapter from sessions with our own patients, the notion of "deserving" food arose repeatedly. Thus food may serve as a treat, or a way of being nice to oneself. Recent evidence suggests that for some people, food is one of a very limited number of pleasurable activities (Doell and Hawkins, 1982; Orbach, 1978). That is, some people have few ways to feel good or be nice to themselves other than by eating treats, often as not forbidden fruits of some kind.

Thus, when internal referents no longer guide behavior—in this case, eating—it begins to be controlled by external factors. When hunger is no longer the signal to eat and satiety does not cause eating to terminate, the stage is set for food, eating, and weight to be used for purposes other than their original physiological ones. For some, food and eating serve psychological functions like those we have just discussed. For others, avoiding food and eating may fill similar psychological needs for a sense of control or a way of reducing negative feelings. Sometimes it is not the actual eating or not eating that is important to the individual, but the effects of eating or not eating on one's weight. Getting slim provides many social reinforcers, as we discussed in chapter 5. Friends and relatives generally encourage one to lose weight and compliment one's "improved," slimmer appearance. Even when people go beyond socially acceptable levels of thinness, so that the compliments cease, being thin gives some women a sense of control or power, not to mention plenty of attention in the form of concern over their health and attempts to get them to eat. For someone who has always felt fairly helpless and unable to dictate the course of her life, the power that excessive thinness can bestow may be seen as an improvement over the status quo, and well worth any discomfort involved. Getting fat, on the other hand, may also have its benefits. As Orbach has pointed out (1978), excess weight helps many women to feel big and powerful in the masculine world of career and business, and enables them to be treated nonsexually, as people rather than merely as potential sexual partners. Excess weight may also provide a sense of having physical space for feelings, both positive and negative (Orbach, 1978), or room for mistakes. As one of our patients put it, "As long as I'm fat I have an excuse when things go wrong. I blame my fat for anything bad that happens to me, including my own mistakes. I feel like if I lose weight I would be perfect—but I would also *have* to be perfect. I couldn't ever make mistakes if I were thin." Being fat may also be a way of punishing oneself, of avoiding a "normal" life, or of opting out of competition with others (Orbach, 1978). The list of ways in which people use their body shape, food, or eating for psychological purposes goes on and on.

What seems to link all of these nonphysiological uses of food, eating, and body shape is an underlying inappropriateness, which may to some extent account for the compulsive, driven quality of these behaviors. Since food is not magical, it cannot make the problems that drive one to eat disappear or even lessen. At best, eating provides one with a temporary distraction from one's worries or insufficiencies. After the eating is over, however, one is faced with both the initial problem and the social stigma of the overweight that will result from continual use of food as an escape. Even those who "get rid" of the excess food by somehow purging their bodies report intense fear until "all the food is gone"—at which point guilt and shame take over. Similarly, those who try to change their body shapes in order to change their lives (or themselves) are usually doomed to disappointment, along with the physical discomfort attendant on attempts to deviate from one's natural weight. Losing or gaining weight tends not to change one's personality, problems, or life to any great degree. The problems must be tackled more directly. Deficiencies in the person cannot be compensated for through surface level alterations in appearance, just as eating or dieting doesn't really alleviate anxiety or depression, or compensate for a lack of pleasure in one's life. The inappropriateness of such an approach to one's troubles makes it inevitable that the approach will not succeed, at least not completely. Those who don't immediately abandon eating or dieting as a problem-solving technique are thus forced to work ever harder at it, accounting for the compulsive, driven quality we have remarked upon. A cycle is set up whereby the person eats (or starves) because of a particular complaint, then eats (or starves) some more because the complaint hasn't gone away, but ultimately eats (or starves) because of a lack of alternative responses coupled with distress over the invasion of one's whole existence by the questions of what, when, and whether to eat. Overeaters and undereaters share a sense that food dominates their lives. If they eat they feel guilty, which sparks off either more eating or a renewed determination not to eat. But since it is impossible to avoid eating altogether, the struggle is self-perpetuating.

Thus far in this chapter we have been talking mostly about people whose eating behavior is pathological or abnormal in a clinical (as opposed to statistical) sense. Although anorexia nervosa and bulimia are becoming increasingly common, they are still relatively rare in the sense that they presumably affect only about 2–12 percent of middle class females between the ages of 10 and 40. Dieting, on the other hand, is considered normal and afflicts at least half of this same population. To what extent does the normal dieter share the inappropriate uses of food and body shape and compulsive behavior patterns of the anorexic or bulimic patient?

As we have shown in chapter 6, dieters exhibit some strange behavior concerning food. Dieters overeat relative to nondieters when they are anxious (Herman and Polivy, 1975) and actually gain weight when they are depressed (Polivy and Herman, 1976). This sounds suspiciously like using food to cope with emotional distress. The repeatedly documented "what-the-hell" effect whereby dieters overeat after eating something fattening (see Herman and Polivy, 1980, for a review) suggests that dieters have lost touch with internal hunger and satiety signals and are eating according to other (probably cognitive) cues. Although the overeating may not reach the proportions of a binge, there is still a sense of its being somehow out of control, or compelled. The dieter would be hard put to say, "What the hell, I broke my diet, but I'll just be a little more stringent the rest of the day and get back to my normal diet tomorrow." Instead, the "what-the-hell" serves as a rationalization for the now inevitable continuance of the lapse. Once an infraction of the dietary limit has occurred, it seems exceedingly difficult for dieters to go back to their restrictions until "a new day" or "a new week" begins, enabling them to start "fresh," from the beginning as it were. Even the normal dieter, then, seems out of touch with internal anchors or referents for behavior. Like the anorexic or bulimic patient, the dieter has had to learn to ignore normal hunger signals, and so eats for reasons other than hunger. The normal dieter is also trying to escape his or her natural weight and to conform instead to some other, "external," standard.

The upshot of such misuse of food and weight seems to be a loss of touch not only with internal signals for behavior, but in some senses with oneself. Inner guides become increasingly unreliable and are abandoned for external ones in areas other than eating. As chapter 7 made clear, dieters do not simply eat in a distorted fashion; their emotional and cognitive reactions are also different from normal (or from those of nondieters). Of course, it may be that it is those people whose inner guides and sense of self are weaker to begin with who are most susceptible to external pressures to diet and change their appearance; but dieting has become so pervasive it seems unlikely that only "weaklings" succumb. Whether or not one's sense of self is weak before dieting begins, it certainly seems to be affected by the dieter mentality once in force. Thus, ordinarily intelligent, effective people begin to question their self-worth if the number on the bathroom scale is higher than it was last week. A presumably normal, nonpathologic friend and professional colleague confided, "I can hardly bear to face the world when the scale reads over 120 pounds. I feel fat, ugly, and worthless. Even one pound above my limit [120 pounds] makes me feel depressed. As long as I weigh 118, I feel fine. At 119 I'm already starting to worry, 120 is worse, and anything over that is panic time. On the other hand, 115 makes me euphoric—at least for the one day it lasts! I feel attractive, lively, and sociable, able to take on anything."

The obsession with slenderness can thus become overwhelming, to the point where one's entire self-image and self-esteem are based on weight. Often this becomes so irrational that minor deviations on the bathroom scale dictate one's outlook: if the "magic number" is low, it is a "good" day, but if it is too high, the day is lost before it begins—more dichotomous thinking. Actual appearance no longer seems to be the primary issue; instead, the goal is to hit the "winning number" on the scale. Intelligence, talent, accomplishments, all pale to insignificance in determining the person's self-esteem next to a digit on a ten-dollar, generally inaccurate, weight-measuring device. Internal values lose their impact when measured up against the external feedback provided by the scale. Small wonder, then, that so many people are so estranged from their own inner workings and feelings and so dependent on outside guides, values, and sources of self-worth. In order to win at this "numbers game" one must embrace dieting and its resultant forfeiture of internal referents.

The comparison of normal dieters and people with eating disorders is thus disturbingly instructive. We have, as a society, tended to regard eating disorders as diseases which may strike anyone—or, if not just anyone, then a certain "vulnerable" section of the population. Dieting, by contrast, is seen as something we *do*, rather than as something that *happens* to us. The difference between eating disorders and normal dieting, however, is not a matter of the difference between a disease and a hobby. Normal dieters may not have, strictly speaking, an eating disorder; but they do display disordered eating. And the similarities between anorexics and bulimics, on the one hand, and dieters, on the other, are not confined to eating. The obsessions underlying disordered eating, the sort of magical thinking that promotes it, the investiture of the self into a particular scale reading—all of these are present in the "normal" dieter. There are, of course, differences in the degree of intensity or drivenness between average dieters and those with full-blown eating disorders. But the patterns themselves are more similar than dissimilar; if we choose to call eating disorders "sick," then we cannot call normal dieting "healthy." The fact that normal dieting is so widespread should not blind us to its dangers: it is a low-grade, popular infection.

In chapters 3, 4, and 5, we discussed the most frequently cited medical, social, and personal/psychological reasons for dieting. We believe the most potent cause of dieting resides in the sociocultural pressures discussed in chapter 5. As we suggested there, the current societal emphasis on thinness seem to contribute to both dieting and disordered eating. The simultaneous cultural fetish with food reflected in the proliferation of specialty/gourmet shops, magazines, and newspaper columns, food faddism ("natural" foods, "organically grown" foods, vegetarianism, and so on), trendy restaurants catering to explicit tastes or even specific courses—doesn't every major city have restaurants that serve only/primarily soups, others known for brunches, and, of course, yet others exclusively for desserts?—and the centering of all social occasions on a meal or course—we meet our friends for lunch, brunch, dinner, coffee, or dessert rather than for conversation—probably helps make binge eating as inevitable a consequence of dieting as rain is a consequence of washing the car. So if one diets for social reasons, one is almost certain to overeat as well. We are again forced to ask, if dieting produces so much discomfort why do so many people persist at it?

Although, as we have spent much of this book showing, it is very unlikely that dieting will accomplish what the dieter hopes it will, two factors probably account for the continued prevalence of dieting in our society. The first is that few people are aware that dieting is unlikely to produce the desired results. There are always some people who are successful at any enterprise, no matter how improbable, and dieting is no exception. There are people who diet successfully, lose as much weight as they want, and keep the weight off. Some of them even seem to adjust to their lowered weight without the kinds of side effects we have documented in chapters 6 and 7. It has even been argued that there are more of these successful dieters than the dismal statistics from weight loss programs would lead us to expect (Schachter, 1982). For some of these successful dieters, improvements occur in other areas of their lives as well. It only takes a few such success stories to spread hope that dieting actually *can* make you thinner, more attractive, more fun to be with, more personable, and an all-round better and happier person. Despite the overwhelming odds against any one person, each individual still believes that he or she is the one who can do it.

The second, probably principal, reason for the persistence of dieting in our society is that it is now such a cultural given that few people ever question why they are doing it or what they actually hope to accomplish, let alone whether or not that goal is being met. Women are "supposed" to be slim, and overweight is "bad" for either sex, so of course one diets to at least some degree. Being on a diet at least some of the time has become the norm, and many people obey the norm almost unquestioningly. They may cite any one or combination of the prevalent "reasons" for dieting, but the basic reason for most people is simply that "one can never be too slim or too rich," so one diets (and works).

In accepting this tenet, a person sacrifices his or her individuality and the unique, personal shape dictated by one's own body. Instead, the person agrees that it is important for one's body to look like a particular general standard. It is not hard to see why adolescents, who are still searching for their own identities and who want above all to be like their peers, are particularly susceptible to this message and correspondingly likely to be dieting (Dwyer, 1973; Dwyer and Mayer, 1970). It is harder to understand why so many adults also have so little self-confidence or self-acceptance. Dieting is tantamount to saying, "I am not 'good' enough as I am, so I will change myself." To the extent that this is not an active decision, it is mindless conformity to a ridiculous and unhealthy cultural practice. To the extent that it is an active decision, it is a refusal to accept oneself. In either case, the lack of internal standards for one's behavior becomes extended to one's eating.

If one has actively decided to diet, a lack of internal referents to guide one's eating may be a small price. If people have chosen dieting, know the risks, but still have confidence that losing weight will help some aspect of their lives, they may be willing to control their eating cognitively and try to ignore or overcome the "side effects" outlined in chapters 6 and 7. It is the person who has been dieting without really thinking about it or making a choice who is most likely to feel compelled and uncomfortable. If such people add up the costs and the benefits dieting has produced thus far in their lives, they might decide that losing weight is not, after all, the answer for them. Is it possible, though, to break out of the pattern of starving and overeating once it has begun? Is it possible to regain contact with one's internal guides to eating and living?

Our experience is that it is possible. A person can learn to use food "naturally" again, that is, simply in response to hunger. But what happens to one's weight when hunger—rather than a cognitive calorie counter—determines eating? If a person eats naturally—that is, eats only when hungry and stops when satisfied—his or her weight seems to return pretty much to its "natural" level. If one has been maintaining a weight below one's true natural weight, eating naturally will cause some weight gain. Surprisingly, though, there are many dieters whose weights are actually at a level above their natural weights, and who thus lose weight when they begin to eat "naturally" again. All the years of starving and overeating as well as the increased use of food for extraneous purposes may have led one's "battle of the bulge" to *increase* the bulge. Becoming a noncombattant may be, for some, the way to beat the bulge. Although most people will weigh more at 50 than they did at 20, their natural weight may still be more acceptable to them and to society's standards than is the elevated weight produced by "unnatural" dieting attempts.

Whether natural weight eating lowers or raises one's weight, it is likely to elevate one's comfort, and perhaps, ultimately, one's self-esteem. Breaking out of the binge–starve cycle (or even its minor variant, the overeat–diet cycle) can also help people feel better about themselves. Rather than continue to let eating (or not eating) and the associated "numbers game" dominate one's daily existence, one can regain control over this aspect of life.

CHAPTER 9

Natural Eating
and Dieting

IF bulimia, anorexia nervosa, and compulsive eating are the results of not accepting oneself, what does it mean *to* accept oneself?

As we have seen, the notion of a natural weight, that is, a range of weights appropriate to each individual, entails that one's own normal weight may not match the cultural ideal; for many, it may not even match the population norm. Most characteristics are distributed throughout the population according to what is known as a "bell-shaped" or "normal" curve. This means that most people are clustered toward the middle, having a moderate amount of the characteristic. As one moves in either direction from this middle (or normal) area, fewer and fewer people are found with progressively larger or smaller amounts of the trait in question. Intelligence or IQ is a frequently used example of a "normally distributed" characteristic. Most people have an IQ of around 100, give or take a few points. This, then, is what is known as "normal intelligence." As we move in either direction from this normal, or most usual, level, we find fewer and fewer people with corresponding IQ levels. Thus, there are fewer people with IQs of either 80 or 120 than with IQs of 100, although there are still substantial numbers at each point. As one moves even further from "normal," the number of people drops more drastically. So there are many fewer people with IQs of 60 or 140 than of 100, or even than 80 or 120. Only a very few people with IQs below 50 or above 150 may be found.

Height is another characteristic distributed in this manner. The population norm has changed over the last century such that both men and women are now taller than their ancestors, on the average. But most people are around average height, say about 65 inches for women and 69 inches for men, plus or minus a couple of inches. Few people deviate from average by 5 inches in either direction for their sex, and people shorter or taller than the norm by as much as 6 or 8 inches are rare, although they obviously do exist. People who deviate even more are often looked upon as abnormal—literally, different from normal—which of course they are, in terms of their height. Except in very extreme cases, though, we are not especially surprised by departures from the norm and, by the same token, we don't expect others to be overly concerned with their own heights or to work to change them.

Weight, or body shape, like height, can be expected to be normally distributed throughout any population, such that most people will cluster around the population average, and fewer and fewer people will have very fat or thin physiques. But there are certainly some people who will "naturally" have such physiques. Also, the "average" weight of the population has increased about 3 to 5 pounds (per inch) over the last 20 years, according to the Metropolitan Life Insurance Company tables. Given that the cultural ideal weight has gotten slimmer over that same 20-year period, many people right at the average weight level for their heights will be above the cultural (and often their own) ideal. People who are only slightly above average (or normal, in the population sense) will be even further from the social ideal. And many people well above both the ideal and the population average will still be at weights that are normal (i.e., natural) for their own bodies. So a person's "natural weight,"—that is, the weight that is normal for, and defended in, that particular person—may or may not be "normal" according to population averages or ideals. Accepting oneself may mean accepting that one does not, or possibly *cannot*, look like the "average" person, let alone the cultural ideal.

What are the limitations imposed by natural weight boundaries? As we discussed in chapter 2, people's natural weight ranges are as variable as any other physical characteristic. Some people have high natural weights; others, for one reason or another, have low natural weights. In either case, these weights are defended biobehaviorally, as we have seen. Moreover, some people have broad ranges which their bodies will tolerate comfortably, whereas others have trouble losing or gaining even 5 pounds. Most people, of course, have an easier time gaining weight than losing it, owing to the traditional evolutionary advantage in being able to store excess food as fat rather than simply wasting it by burning it or excreting it. Obviously, we are all descended from people who were able to survive periodic famines, and most of us have inherited to some degree the ability to store at least some of our extra food. It is more difficult, though, to lose weight, since our bodies (unlike our cars) seem to become automatically more fuel efficient when faced with a threat of a shortage. That may be why more people become obese than anorexic. If one wanted to work out one's psychological problems by altering one's appearance, clearly it would generally be easier to round out curves with more fat than to flatten them through weight loss. The more usual desire, though, is to lose pounds and to keep them off. Regardless of one's motives—whether a simple desire to improve one's appearance and achieve a more socially desirable image, or a more complex need to resolve psychological problems—the ease with which one can alter one's body shape depends to a great extent upon how flexible one's natural weight boundaries are. People with rigidly defended upper and/or lower boundaries will have more trouble going beyond them than will people with more loosely defended boundaries. Alternatively, people with broader natural weight ranges have more room to move their weights around comfortably than do those with smaller ranges.

A key word in the preceding sentence is *comfortably*. Regardless of how confined one's natural weight range is, or how rigidly defended its boundaries are, it is still theoretically possible to move beyond those boundaries. By eating a lot more than one's body requires and moving around as little as possible, most (but not all) people will be able to raise their weight at least somewhat above their natural upper boundaries. Similarly, by eating very little—for some people this may mean next to nothing at all—and moving around and/or exercising as much as possible, most people can lower their weights below their natural lower boundaries, as countless anorexia nervosa patients have demonstrated. The key issue, however, is how comfortable one is likely to be while maintaining a weight above or below one's natural weight range. The amount of overeating or starving necessary to maintain such unnatural weights may make for an extremely uncomfortable existence. Moreover, as we discussed earlier, there are likely to be other costs beyond the direct need to eat until bloated or starve until faint. As we discussed in chapters 3 and 4, many of the medical problems usually associated with obesity may actually be a result of deviating from one's natural weight. Most diseases thought to be due to overweight can more accurately be accounted for by overeating alone, or by dieting, or by a combination of the two that results in "yo-yoing." And apart from the medical problems—which occur only after years of abuse to the body, and tend to be ignored until they happen—there are the side effects of dieting reviewed in chapters 6 and 7. Dieters tend to be more emotional, more distractible, and generally more upset than nondieters. They also become more likely to eat (and overeat) in just about every kind of situation studied thus far. More ominously, many dieters apparently become periodic bingers or bulimics, whose lives ultimately revolve around alternately starving and stuffing themselves.

The penalties for forcing one's body outside its natural weight limits may be acceptable, though, if one gets enough reward for one's new physique. Since, as we discussed in chapter 5, attractiveness is an important attribute in our society, and current cultural standards call slenderness attractive, there are often social rewards for weight loss. At the very least, people often harvest praise and compliments on their "improved" appearance. (However, many people tell anyone they haven't seen in a while that they look well and "must have lost weight," whether this is true or not. The fact that it has virtually become a mere social custom may mitigate the value of such a "compliment" to some more wary recipients.) Although we argue throughout this book that weight loss is not a panacea, and will not necessarily produce the desired consequences even for those who are successful at it, there are some people who *do* realize their goals simply by losing weight. And, as Schachter (1982) has found, there are many people who decide to lose weight and simply do so. These people were able to lose weight on their own, and they maintained their lowered weight for several years. For such people, the costs of weight loss may prove worthwhile.

In conjunction with Schachter's findings, it is interesting to note that his estimate of the proportion of overweight dieters likely eventually to be successful at losing weight is approximately 62 to 72 percent. This figure corresponds rather closely with estimates of the percentage of adult onset (or what we would consider "above natural weight") obese persons in the overweight population (70 percent adult onset versus 30 percent juvenile onset; see Milich, 1975). This suggests to us that Schachter's demonstration that obesity is not as resistant to cure as most weight loss therapy studies indicate may be highlighting the difference between weight loss in the service of return to natural weight (by adult onset obese people who gained over time to more than their natural weights) and attempted weight loss in defiance of natural weight (those remaining 30 to 40 percent who were always overweight—or juvenile onset obese—and always unsuccessful at long-term weight loss). For adult onset obese people—presumably the vast majority of the overweight population—their excess weight represents "unnatural" accretions for whatever reasons (changes in eating patterns, emotionally induced overeating, and so on). This weight in excess of the body's natural weight is reasonably amendable to reduction, since the body is not disposed to maintain the extra weight. Thus, for 60–70 percent of overweight people, weight loss may not always be all that difficult, and maintenance of the lowered weight simply requires that one refrain from prolonged overeating. For the other 30 percent of the overweight population, however, weight loss involves eluding the body's defenses of its natural weight, which seems to demand chronic semistarvation. Not surprisingly, few of the juvenile onset, "naturally" overweight people are able to manage this constant vigilance and become dieting success statistics.

For many such people, the penalties for defying their natural weights will be much more severe than can be offset by any benefits that may be derived. This net failure may reflect the strength of the physical or emotional side effects accompanying weight loss, or the fact that the expected benefits don't materialize. For even more people, attempts to defy their natural weights will simply prove unsuccessful. Such people either will not lose as much weight as they hope to or will be unable to maintain a lowered weight long enough to derive any benefits from slenderness. It is sad but true that, to paraphrase Albert Stunkard, most such people who try to lose weight will fail, and most who succeed will rapidly regain their lost pounds. If such people were more aware ahead of time of the difficulties (both physical and psychological) of losing weight and keeping that weight from returning, they might be less deterred by them and ultimately less disappointed.

We hope that after reading this book, at least some people will be not only more aware of the problems they face if they decide to lose weight, but also more skeptical about the need to do so. For those people who have been dieting for years without really thinking about what they are doing and what they hope to accomplish by it, we have tried to bring forward these and similar questions. Our goal in writing this book has been, at least partially, to question the prevailing view that overweight is bad and dangerous whereas dieting and weight loss are good and healthy. We also question the whole notion that one's body shape should be of major import in one's life, especially for people who are really not "abnormal" (i.e., different from normal or average, for themselves or the population in general). What we would like to promote is an acceptance of individual differences in body shape, just as differences in hem length are now tolerated. Instead of mindless acceptance of an unhealthy cultural ideal, which is probably unmaintainable for many, and unlikely to produce a great deal of happiness even in those capable of achieving and maintaining it, we propose that people try to return to their natural weights, and relegate eating to its more natural place in their lives.

How does a person know what his or her natural weight is? There is as yet no physiological measure that directly indicates a person's natural weight range or body weight set point. Likewise, there are no objective tests for determining how stringently or loosely one's weight range boundaries are defended. This means that, at least for the present, the only way to determine what a person's natural weight should be is empirically—that is, by having them eat naturally (i.e., for hunger, but not for other reasons) until their weight stabilizes. A rough estimate of natural weight can probably be made if during adulthood the person ever maintained a fairly stable weight without artificial restrictions or dieting, or without unnecessary overeating beyond the body's needs. Some adjustment has to be made for increasing age—weight tends to rise a bit every decade after maturity is reached—but one's natural weight is probably within 5 pounds of one's weight at age 21, *if* one were eating normally at that time. People who have been dieters "all their lives" may not be able to estimate easily what their natural weight is, as dieting can put them below or above this level. Paradoxically, as we have seen, some perennial dieters actually weigh more than they would if they had never dieted. Because dieting often makes people more conservative metabolically—usually the body begins to use what food it does receive more efficiently—and seems frequently to engender the eating of large (often excessive) quantities of foods, on periodic binges or disinhibited "what-the-hell" episodes, the end result may be a weight considerably higher than the weight that initiated the decision to diet. Moreover, when people regain weight that they have lost on a diet, they often gain more than they originally lost. In the conscientious objector starvation study (Keys et al., 1950) which we discussed in previous chapters, the subjects regained to a level slightly above their original weight, and a higher percentage of their refed weight was fat than before they were starved. It is thus not as crazy as it seems to say that dieting may make people overweight.

This obviously calls into question the whole notion of dieting. Most people think of dieting as some form of caloric restriction resulting in weight loss. As we have tried to explain in this book, though, it is not that simple. Dieting, or being on a diet, means different things to different people. For some people dieting involves eating the same things they normally do, but cutting down the amounts. Others diet by eliminating or cutting down on certain kinds of foods. Still others shift their eating patterns completely, eating only a limited variety of foods, sometimes in specific combinations, orders, or time periods. Any of these dieting techniques can be done moderately or very stringently. Even someone pursuing the wisest plan of simply cutting down amounts but eating all foods can cut down to an insufficient number of calories (below 1,200 or so), whereas the person on a limited number of foods may nonetheless choose a well-balanced (though necessarily repetitious) combination in sufficient quantities to ensure a healthy weight loss of no more than 1–2 pounds per week. When we say that dieting causes overweight, then, it is important to specify what kind of dieting we mean.

As far as we are concerned, the evidence reviewed in this book suggests that any dieting that involves feeling deprived, or deviating far from one's natural weight, will have sequelae or side effects. The more drastic the caloric and nutritional restrictions (i.e., the smaller the variety and quantity of foods eaten), the more serious the potential side effects seem to be. The reverse, however, is also true. The more drastic the overeating, and deviation above one's natural weight, the more harm (both physical and emotional) one is likely to suffer.

What does this mean for the countless chronic dieters in our society? How can they break the cycle of starving and stuffing themselves, and bring their weight and eating back under control? The answer, we believe, is to return to their natural weight and natural eating. In order to do this, one must go on what we call the "natural weight *un*diet." This involves undoing the cognitive or psychological patterns that dieting established.

The first step is to become reacquainted with the feelings from the body that signal hunger and satiety. People who eat their meals at regular hours every day tend to feel hungry as those mealtimes approach. Another way to recognize hunger is to stop before eating and ask, "How do I feel right now? Do I really want this food? Do I need something in my stomach or is it only my mouth which craves a particular taste?" It is important to distinguish between hunger, the body's physiological need for food, and appetite, a psychologically instigated desire for a particular taste or sensation in the mouth or even the stomach. (Some people want their stomachs to feel quite full or even somewhat bloated.) People who have difficulty identifying hunger might find it easier if they ate nothing but three or four well-balanced, tasty meals each day at the same times every day for a week or so. This should condition the physiological signals of hunger to occur at those mealtimes.

Satiety, or the point at which hunger has been satisfied, may be even more difficult to identify. Many people were brought up as members of the "clean plate club," and believe that they are not finished (or sated) until their plates are empty. At home, where one can serve oneself small or moderate portions and seconds as needed, this may not be a major problem. However, restaurants seldom gear their portion sizes to the particular nutritional needs of individual diners, and at dinner parties hosts often overestimate their guests' appetites. Learning to stop eating when hunger has been satisfied is therefore a crucial—and often difficult—step. The literature on behavior modification offers some helpful techniques for learning to recognize satiety. Putting down one's fork between bites and sipping water frequently during the meal slow down one's eating and give opportunities for thinking about whether or not more food is necessary. It is also very helpful to stop eating for a full minute halfway and three-quarters of the way through the meal. During these "rests" one should concentrate on how one's stomach feels and on whether one is actually still hungry. If the answer is not a clear "yes," the remaining food should be wrapped up and put away. Often the mere reassurance that the food is still available is sufficient to stave off cravings brought on more by the mind than the body. Another technique is to put only two-thirds or three-quarters of one's usual portion onto the plate, treating the rest as seconds to be eaten if one is still hungry. Finally, some people may need to actually interrupt their meal with another activity, returning to the table only if they find they are still hungry after another 15 minutes or so. Initially, at least, it may help to cover any extra food not eaten at meals and put it away for later. Again, this provides assurance that the food is still available in the event that one gets hungry before the next meal. Several of our patients have been surprised to find that they never seem to want (let alone need) the "extra" food they store this way.

For the overeater who eats more than is needed simply from habit ("that's how much I've always eaten") or, like Sir Edmund Hillary, because it's there ("I eat until my plate—or the pot—is clean"), such techniques usually prove effective. The undieter soon learns how much food his or her body really requires and can begin to eat naturally. For those caught in the starve-or-stuff cycle of chronic dieting or binge eating, these techniques may not be sufficient to overcome the attractions of food. To binge eaters, food often comes to represent comfort, companionship, a time filler for empty hours, a way to vent otherwise inexpressible emotions, the means for filling an internal void, or a special treat, something tantalizing yet forbidden. Such people must learn to devalue (the now overvalued) food. Its magical, symbolic qualities must be eliminated so that it can be treated naturally again. This process is often exceptionally difficult, and some people may in effect be hopelessly addicted to at least an occasional "food fix." The occasional binge need not drastically affect one's weight, however; nor is it the same as the obsession with food and daily binges that many dieters currently experience.

How, then, can the committed dieter–gorger learn to eat naturally? Since food has become such a central and critical component of the dieter's emotional life, it is necessary to seek some substitute for at least some of the extra functions food has been fulfilling. Since food seems to represent for most dieters a way of being nicer to (or treating) themselves, other, less self-destructive treats need to be identified. The more such treats are available, the more likely that the dieter will be able to turn to one of these alternatives rather than food when the need arises. The specific alternatives chosen are of necessity idiosyncratic and personal, but some things have been endorsed by several of our (ex-)patients. Some self-enhancing treats mentioned to us include bubble baths, walks, visits to a masseur, health club, or beauty salon, a phone call to a friend (long distance, perhaps), and gifts to oneself. Small gifts—special skin cream, bath oil, hair ornaments, cologne, handmade soap, small articles of clothing, knickknacks, pens, and so on—can either be bought spontaneously when the occasion demands or kept on hand (gift-wrapped, of course) for late night urges. Larger gifts can be saved for and savored in advance—a trip, a stereo, or special clothes can be the final treat which has in a sense already been enjoyed each time one has put aside some of the money to pay for it. Another treat may simply be time taken from a busy schedule to relax or be by oneself, reading or listening to music (which may involve buying new records or tapes), or even just taking time to groom oneself better. Daytime and late night activities must both be included, of course, and it is often useful to have at least some that are incompatible with eating (like exercising or leaving the house).

Having suitable alternative treats is essential, but usually not sufficient in and of itself. Food has often become so mystically alluring that it is necessary for the bingers to see more graphically the power that food holds for them. Accordingly, we have found it useful to help our patients to become aware of various aspects of their addiction. One such issue centers on getting patients to learn to throw food away. For many, the mere idea of wasting food seems almost sacrilegious. Behavior therapists frequently recommend that their overweight patients leave a bite or two on their plates. We go a step further and urge our patients to take those remaining bites and personally throw them in the garbage. For some people, this requires a Herculean effort (and it is amazing how often one can "forget" to do such a simple, trivial assignment). After this simple task has been mastered (which may take weeks), for some patients it may be necessary to make the point more directly. For these patients, we have devised the "toilet binge." This involves having the binger buy the food for a typical binge, bring it home, and throw it into the toilet (since this is where it will eventually wind up one way or the other). The food should be broken into bite-sized pieces and crumbled with the hands before being thrown into the toilet to keep the exercise as similar to the reality as possible. This "skip the middleman" technique usually drives home the point—food in excess of the body's needs is essentially being poured down the toilet (or onto one's hips). One of our patients described the effect this exercise had on her as follows:

> I started with the cookies. The oatmeal ones crumbled easily and I threw them in. The chocolate ones were a bit messier and my hands got smeared with chocolate. Next went a bag of Cheesies, and the concoction in the toilet started to look pretty nauseating. My hands were also pretty awful—brown and orange. What really did it for me, though, was the quart of ice cream. I usually buy the cheapest brand for my binges since by the time I get to the ice cream I don't really notice how it tastes. I started spooning the stuff into the toilet, and I noticed that it wasn't melting. I kept spooning and spooning and the stuff just floated around in little blobs. I looked at this scummy mess and said, "Is this what I've

been putting into my stomach, into my body?" and I wanted to throw up, even though I hadn't eaten anything. I realized that this wasn't being nice to myself, this was punishing myself. I'm finally starting to realize I deserve better than this!

The toilet binge is thus a powerful technique in several respects for helping binge eaters to become aware of what they are doing to themselves when they stuff themselves with unnatural quantities of food. (We tried garbage can binges initially, but our patients were not as powerfully affected, and some had trouble not going back and eating some of the food later!) Not only does it emphasize the excessiveness and wastefulness of the eating, but it provides a graphic depiction of the unappetizing, unhealthy substances being stuffed into one's stomach during a binge. Most bingers we have encountered find this an enlightening experience.

Although these exercises may not immediately induce a conversion to natural eating and a rejection of binge eating or even mild overeating, they seem to make such a conversion more feasible. We cannot emphasize enough that binge eating is a pernicious and painful problem, which is not cured magically and quickly. We have found the techniques we have described useful in helping binge eaters to become reacquainted with their bodies and their natural eating patterns.

Once hunger and satiety are again controlling food intake, many people—whether initially binge eaters or normal dieters —find they eat less than they previously did. Body weight should begin to stabilize at a level comfortable for the individual, his or her natural weight. At that point, one should be able to eat any food whenever one wants to—providing, of course, that one eats only when hungry, stopping as soon as the initial hunger is satisfied. This means not stuffing oneself until uncomfortably full or bloated. For many people, satiety has generally meant this sensation of fullness rather than the elimination of hunger. Eating naturally involves stopping well before any discomfort would begin. So we are not advocating that people eat all they want of whatever they desire in the usual sense. It is crucial first to learn the distinction between "wanting" (for whatever psychological reasons) and "needing" (physiologically). We are thus saying that people should eat as much as they *need* (to be comfortably satisfied) of whatever food they want. This is the crux of the natural weight undiet.

As indicated, there should be no forbidden food. Even if one is trying to lose weight, small portions of high calorie foods (e.g., one scoop of ice cream, one doughnut, or a slice or two of pizza) should be incorporated into one's *weekly* diet. Thinking in terms of a week rather than a day, as well as allowing all types of food, helps to avoid the diet mentality that produces eating binges. One nondiet meal isn't enough to ruin a whole week's worth of undieting, so there is no need to continue overeating after a "transgression." Allowing all foods also reduces the need to find excuses for breaking the undiet (in order to get at the "forbidden fruits"). Any eating, or even weight loss promoting regime should be comfortable enough so that the undieter (a) doesn't feel deprived, (b) is able to incorporate occasional splurges without feeling guilty, and (c) can continue to eat in this manner for a lifetime (since that will most likely be necessary to maintain losses to or, for those who decide they still prefer a lower weight, below natural weight levels).

Any behavioral change techniques that will make it easier to be comfortable with a normal caloric intake should also be incorporated into one's new eating style. Leaving the dining area immediately after a meal rather than sitting over the leftovers helps put food out of mind, as does storing leftovers in opaque containers, or throwing them away altogether (a difficult task for many, as we have mentioned, but better than throwing them away into one's own body). Low calorie, nutritious snacks like fresh fruit or vegetables should be kept handy and ready to eat (i.e., cleaned and cut in snack-sized pieces). A sensible program of moderate, regular exercise may not only increase the expenditure of calories, but help the person feel more fit and vigorous as well. And the alleged problem of exercise increasing hunger—and thus canceling out its own benefits—is simply not a problem for most of us. It's only at "lumberjack" levels of exercise that hunger increases; for most of us, regular exercise—especially before meals—is as likely as not to *decrease* appetite. Similarly, a cup of warm broth or a small salad at the start of a meal often helps to reduce the amount of food one needs to eat at that meal. This can help satisfy a person who can only have one slice of pizza for lunch instead of an accustomed two or more. The important point is that although returning to natural weight may for some involve a certain amount of deprivation and/or discomfort, these should be minimized in order to forestall an all-or-nothing diet-or-gorge attitude. Furthermore, a nutritionally balanced diet of *at least* 1,200–1,500 calories a day (and most undieters will find they need more like 2,000) will help prevent many of the dieting-induced health problems discussed in chapter 4. Finally, any weight change attempt should be preceded by a medical check-up, and the maximal weekly weight loss sought, even in a reduction back to natural weight, should not exceed 1–2 pounds. As we pointed out in chapter 4, and as is important to reiterate here, undereating seems to cause almost as many medical problems as overeating. For many people, natural eating is a lot more difficult than it sounds. Certain foods have for so long been considered taboo that eating even a small quantity of them triggers thoughts that ultimately lead to overeating or even a true binge. It is for this reason that we have stressed that no food should be forbidden. As the experiments we described in chapter 6 amply demonstrated, it is as often as not simply the idea that one has "blown the diet" or overeaten—by eating some "nondiet" food like chocolate, cake, or ice cream—that causes real overeating. Moreover, the frustration of being denied a favorite "treat" food can contribute to a half-unconscious desire to have an excuse for "pigging out" and eating the treat. This sort of self-sabotage is eliminated by making every food allowable. If there is no such thing as "breaking" or "blowing" the diet, there is no longer any basis for the "what-the-hell" effect. Furthermore, as we saw in chapter 7, people who are eating naturally will be less prone to the sorts of emotional upsets that trigger overeating in chronic dieters.

While we are on the subject of self-sabotage, we should mention another problem many undieters will face—namely, social sabotage. We have been discussing the natural weight undiet as if the only one involved were the undieter. This is true only up to a point. Other people in the environment exert a major influence over what and even how much an individual eats. As most dieters can attest, that influence is not always helpful. For the undieter, it can be even worse. Most people —even dinner party hosts—will accept "I'm on a diet" as an excuse for avoiding seconds or dessert. It is harder to explain the undiet, however. If you ate the béarnaise sauce at dinner —because you were truly hungry and that was what you wanted —your host may find it hard to accept that you are too full for dessert, and that your undiet insists that you stop eating. You may find yourself with a heaping plate of seconds or dessert or other food you don't want or need before you can say "undiet." It is difficult in our society, where a clean plate is a compliment to the chef and a morsel left an insult, to learn that one does not *have* to eat whatever one is given. A host so insensitive as to ignore the guest's expressed wishes doesn't deserve to be complimented with a clean plate—especially at the undieter's expense.

Western society may not be unusual in the emphasis it places on food during social occasions. Sharing food is probably a universal means of expressing friendship and good feelings. A birthday party without cake and ice cream, or other appropriate culinary delights, depending on the age of the celebrants, would be a second-rate affair. It has gotten to the point, however, where any socializing seems to require refreshment. Whenever friends meet, they meet for breakfast, lunch, brunch, tea, coffee, a drink, cocktails, dinner, or (again) coffee. If friends drop by for a visit, it is a social solecism not to at least offer refreshments. The undieter is thus under a lot of social pressure to eat at times when he or she may not be hungry. Saying "I just ate, thanks," or "Just coffee for me; I'm not really hungry" is often not as easy as it sounds. And, if everyone else is having pie à la mode, the undieter may feel a bit deprived drinking iced tea. In such instances, it is better to take the pie à la mode and eat only a few bites—enough to satisfy but not stuff. One shouldn't feel that money is being wasted because the food is left on the plate (assuming some unrestrained friend doesn't finish it). That food was excess—waste—anyway; eating it doesn't make the money better spent!

The kinds of social pressures to eat that we have just mentioned are probably the most common, as well as the easiest to combat. More insidious is the sort of sabotage practised by jealous dieter friends or relatives, or by those who otherwise prefer their nearest and dearest to remain overweight. These saboteurs couch their pressure to overeat as concern for the undieter's health, welfare, or enjoyment. One of our patients described her spouse's concern that she was eating less now that her undieting had helped her to stop overeating when she wasn't hungry.

> He urged me to have special treats ("Just this once won't hurt"), kept offering me tidbits from his own plate ("I know you love this, so why don't *you* have it"), and requested that I join him in excess snacking or overeating ("Come on, have some—don't make me eat alone"). Yet, for years he had teased me about my excess weight and my inability to lose it, while bragging about the ease with which he could take off a few pounds whenever he wanted to. And what really got me was that he *could* do it, without seeming to suffer! Every time I gave up on my latest diet and ate something fattening, he would shake his head and look disgusted. He would say something like, "Do you really *need* that?" I would stop, but as soon as his back was turned I'd sneak back and eat twice as much just to show him or something. He's stopped that now that I'm "undieting"—I told him my doctor said I should get used to eating all kinds of foods. Now, though, it's like he doesn't like it that I'm losing the weight. He tries to make me eat more and more, and sometimes it's easier to give in than to examine whether I really do want to eat it.

As weight loss therapists have observed for years, it is often the case that the spouse, friends, or family of an overweight person prefer that person to remain overweight, despite what they may say. The patient we quoted above finally brought her husband in for a few therapy sessions with her, so that his feelings about her weight could be explored. While this was an extreme example, it is all too often true that *someone* in the overweight person's life either wants that person to remain overweight (and will work actively to that end) or comments unduly on what and how much he or she eats and weighs. The undieter must therefore be prepared to deal with such interference from others. The "helpful" person who says "Should you really be eating pizza?" can be just as destructive as the fat friend who urges the undieter to overeat. Whether such people are trying to help or hinder the undieter at losing weight, they must be tactfully asked not to interfere. Undieting involves getting back in touch with, and accepting, one's own body. Those committed to seeing the undieter either thinner or fatter may not accept this decision to accept oneself however one is. For some people, however, a basic explanation of undieting and its purpose will be sufficient. Others might simply have to be told to mind their own business (their rudeness in worrying so much about what someone else is eating might reflect an inability to let others manage their own lives). In any case, the undieter must recognize that one's own eating behavior is affected by other people, either wittingly or unwittingly. Influences counterproductive to undieting must be identified and prevented from manipulating the undieter's food intake.

Our natural weight undiet is obviously intended for those who have decided that they do not want to pay the costs of weighing less or more than their natural weight, who would prefer to try to accept themselves and be comfortable even if that turns out to mean weighing more than is fashionable. On the other hand, we recognize that, given prevailing cultural pressures, some people may decide that their appearance is important enough to them to justify the discomforts of dieting. We would like to reemphasize for them our contention that dieting may result not only in discomfort, but in a *higher* weight. Those whose dieting attempts have been successful in producing a stable lower weight may be willing to continue to accept any side effects they are experiencing. Those who find their successes continually interrupted by bouts of disordered eating and/or weight gain might be better advised to reconsider the costs of those successes.

One of the messages of this book is that dieters should be aware of the hazards they face. These include negative side effects of weight loss and the frustrations of the attempt(s), as well as the physical and psychological obstacles to deviations from natural weight. We have attempted to raise questions about the whole enterprise of losing weight/being thin in order to make people aware of what they are doing. We have tried to help people to discover their own motivations and make a conscious choice about whether or not to continue. We have tried to examine what people hope to get from dieting, and what they are likely actually to attain. For those who choose to be thin, we hope we have clarified the problems to be faced. Deviating from natural weight is difficult because it is in some sense unnatural, and, as we have been told so often, "It's not nice to fool Mother Nature." Indeed, dieters must ask themselves: Who's fooling whom? The accumulating evidence that dieting may derange one's eating, disconnect the natural linkages between mind and body, and even accelerate the very weight gains that are most dreaded must make us wonder whether, by abandoning dieting, we might not be more likely to regain our lost selves than our lost weight.

References

Abraham, S.; Collins, G.; and Nordsieck, M. 1971. Relationship of child-hood weight status to morbidity in adults. *H.S.M.H.A. Health Reports* 86:273–84.

Abramson, E. E., and Wunderlich, R. A. 1972. Anxiety, fear, and eating: A test of the psychosomatic concept of obesity. *Journal of Abnormal Psychology* 79:317–21.

Air Force Diet. 1960. Toronto: Air Force Diet Publishers.

Angel, A., and Roncari, D. A. K. 1978. Medical complications of obesity. *Canadian Medical Association Journal* 119:1408–11.

Atkins, R. C. 1972. *Dr. Atkins's diet revolution: The high calorie way to stay thin forever.* New York: David McKay, Inc.

Baird, I. M.; Parsons, R. L.; and Howard, A. N. 1974. Clinical and metabolic studies of chemically defined diets in the management of obesity. *Metabolism* 23:645–57.

Ball, M. F.; Canary, J. J.; and Kyle, L. H. 1967. Comparative effects of caloric restriction and total starvation on body composition in obesity. *Annals of Internal Medicine* 67:60–67.

Beck, S. B.; Ward-Hull, C. I.; and McLear, P. M. 1976. Variables related

References

to women's somatic preferences for the male and female body. *Journal of Personality and Social Psychology* 34:1200–10.

Beller, A. S. 1978. *Fat and thin: a natural history of obesity.* New York: Farrar, Straus & Giroux.

Bennett, W., and Gurin, J. 1982. *The dieter's dilemma.* New York: Basic Books.

Berscheid, E., and Walster, E. 1974. Physical attractiveness. In *Advances in experimental social psychology, vol. 7,* ed. L. Berkowitz, pp. 158–215. New York: Academic Press.

Bistrian, B. R., and Sherman, M. 1978. Results of the treatment of obesity with a protein-sparing modified fast. *International Journal of Obesity* 2:143–48.

Bistrian, B. R.; Winterer, J.; Blackburn, G. L.; Young, V.; and Sherman, M. 1977. Effect of a protein-sparing diet and brief fast on nitrogen metabolism in mildly obese subjects. *Journal of Laboratory and Clinical Medicine* 89:1030–35.

Bjurlf, P. 1959. Atherosclerosis and body build with special reference to size and number of subcutaneous fat cells. *Acta Medica Scandinavica,* supplement #349, pp. 1–99.

Bloom, W. L. 1959. Fasting as an introduction to the treatment of obesity. *Metabolism* 8:214–20.

Boskind-Lodahl, M. 1976. Cinderella's stepsisters: a feminist perspective on anorexia nervosa and bulimia. *Signs: Journal of Women in Culture and Society* 2:342–56.

Bradley, P. J. 1980. Obesity, diet and coronary heart disease: A dissenting view. *Medical Journal of Australia* 1:277–85.

Branch, C. H. H., and Eurman, L. J. 1980. Social attitudes toward patients with anorexia nervosa. *American Journal of Psychiatry* 137:631–32.

Bray, G. A. 1976. *The obese patient.* Toronto: Saunders.

Brosin, H. W. 1954. The psychiatric aspects of obesity. *Journal of the American Medical Association* 155:1238–39.

Bruch, H. 1973. *Eating disorders.* New York: Basic Books.

Bruch, H. 1978. *The golden cage.* Cambridge, Mass.: Harvard University Press.

Cabanac, M.; Duclaux, R.; and Spector, N. H. 1971. Sensory feedback in regulation of body weight: Is there a ponderostat? *Nature* 229:125–27.

Casper, R. C.; Eckert, E. D.; Halmi, K. A.; Goldberg, S. C.; and Davis, J. M. 1980. Bulimia—Its incidence and clinical importance in patients with anorexia nervosa. *Archives of General Psychiatry* 37:1030–35.

References

Cavallo-Perin, P.; Sorbo, G.; Morra, A.; Pagani, A.; Taaliaferro, V.; and Lenti, G. 1981. Correlation between obesity and other risk factors for coronary heart disease in a group of 4124 volunteers. In *Obesity pathogenesis and treatment*, eds. G. Enzi, G. Crepaldi, G. Pozza, and A. E. Renold, pp. 297–303. New York: Academic Press.

Council on Foods and Nutrition, American Medical Association. 1973. A critique of low-carbohydrate ketogenic weight reduction regimens—A review of Dr. Atkins's diet revolution. *Journal of the American Medical Association* 224:1415–19.

Cubberley, P. T.; Polster, S. A.; and Schulman, C. L. 1965. Lactic acidosis and death after the treatment of obesity by fasting. *New England Journal of Medicine* 272:628–30.

Dermer, M., and Thiel, D. 1975. When beauty may fail. *Journal of Personality and Social Psychology* 31:1168–76.

Dion, K. 1972. Physical attractiveness and evaluation of children's transgressions. *Journal of Personality and Social Psychology* 24:207–13.

Dion, K.; Berscheid, E.; and Walster, E. 1972. What is beautiful is good. *Journal of Personality and Social Psychology* 24:285–90.

Doell, S. R., and Hawkins, R. C. 1982. Pleasures and pounds: An exploratory study. *Addictive Behaviors* 7:65–69.

Drenick, E. J. 1979. Definition and health consequences of morbid obesity. *Surgical Clinics of North America* 59:963–76.

Drenick, E. J., and Alvarez, L. C. 1971. Neutropenia in prolonged fasting. *American Journal of Clinical Nutrition* 24:859–63.

Drenick, E. J.; Stanley, T. M.; and Wills, C. E. 1981. Renal damage after intestinal bypass. *International Journal of Obesity* 5:501–8.

Drenick, E. J.; Swendseid, M. E.; Blahd, W. H.; and Tuttle, S. G. 1964. Prolonged starvation as treatment for severe obesity. *Journal of the American Medical Association* 187:140–45.

Duncan, G. G.; Cristofori, F. C.; Yue, J. K.; and Murthy, M. S. J. 1964. The control of obesity by intermittent fasts. *Medical Clinics of North America* 48:1359–72.

Duncan, G. G.; Duncan, T. G.; Schless, G. L.; and Cristofori, F. C. 1965. Contraindications and therapeutic results of fasting in obese patients. *Annals of the New York Academy of Science* 131:632–36.

Dwyer, J. T. 1973. Psychosexual aspects of weight control and dieting behavior in adolescents. *Medical Aspects of Human Sexuality*, March, pp. 82–108.

References

Dwyer, J. T.; Feldman, J. J.; and Mayer, J. 1967. Adolescent dieters: Who are they? *American Journal of Clinical Nutrition* 20:1045–56.

Dwyer, J. T.; Feldman, J. J.; and Mayer, J. 1970. The social psychology of dieting. *Journal of Health and Social Behavior* 11:269–87.

Dwyer, J. T.; Feldman, J. J.; Seltzer, C. C.; and Mayer, J. 1969. Adolescent attitudes toward weight and appearance. *Journal of Nutrition Education* 1:14–19.

Dwyer, J. T., and Mayer, J. 1970. Potential dieters: Who are they? *Journal of American Dietetic Association* 56:510–14.

Ely, R. J.; Goolkasian, G.; Frost, R. O.; and Blanchard, F. A. 1979. Dieting, depression, and eating behavior. Paper presented at the 1979 Annual Meeting of the American Psychological Association, New York.

Esses, V.; Herman, C. P.; and Polivy, J. 1982. A boundary interpretation of "counter-regulation." Unpublished manuscript, University of Toronto.

Feinstein, A. R. 1960. The treatment of obesity: an analysis of methods, results and factors which influence success. *Journal of Chronic Disease* 11:349–93.

Franklin, J. S., Schiele, B. C.; Brozek, J.; and Keys, A. 1948. Observations in human behavior in experimental starvation and rehabilitation. *Journal of Clinical Psychology* 4:28–45.

Garfinkel, P. E., and Garner, D. M. 1982. *Anorexia nervosa: A multi-dimensional perspective.* New York: Brunner/Mazel.

Garfinkel, P. E.; Moldofsky, H.; and Garner, D. M. 1980. The heterogeneity of anorexia nervosa—bulimia as a distinct subgroup. *Archives of General Psychiatry* 37:1036–40.

Garfinkel, P. E.; Moldofsky, H.; Garner, D. M.; Stancer, H. C.; and Coscina, D. V. 1978. Body awareness in anorexia nervosa: disturbances in "body image" and "satiety." *Psychosomatic Medicine* 40:487–98.

Garner, D. M.; Garfinkel, P. E.; Schwartz, D.; and Thompson, M. 1980. Cultural expectations of thinness in women. *Psychological Reports* 47:483–91.

Garnett, E. S.; Barnard, D. L.; Ford, J.; Goodbody, R. A.; and Woodenhouse, M. A. 1969. Gross fragmentation of cardiac myofibrils after therapeutic starvation for obesity. *The Lancet,* no. i, 914–16.

Genuth, S. M., Castro, J. H., and Vertes, V. 1978. Weight reduction in obesity by outpatient semi starvation. *Journal of the American Medical Association* 230:987–91.

References

Gilliland, I. C. 1968. Total fasting in the treatment of obesity. *Postgraduate Medical Journal* 44:58–61.

Glucksman, M. L., and Hirsch, J. 1968. The response of obese patients to weight reduction, II: A qualitative evaluation of behavior. *Psychosomatic Medicine* 30:359–72.

Goldblatt, P. B., Moore, M. E., and Stunkard, A. J. 1965. Social factors in obesity. *Journal of the American Medical Association* 192:1039–44.

Grinker, J. 1973. Behavioral and metabolic consequences of weight reduction. *Journal of the American Dietetic Association* 62:30–34.

Hamburger, W. W. 1951. Emotional aspects of obesity. *Medical Clinics of North America* 35:483–99.

Hampton, M. C.; Hueneman, R. L.; Shapiro, L. R.; Mitchell, B. W.; and Behnke, A. R. 1966. A longitudinal study of gross body composition and body conformation and their association with food and activity in a teenage population: Anthropometric evaluation of a body build. *American Journal of Clinical Nutrition* 19:422–35.

Harrison, M. T., and Harden, R. M. 1966. The long-term value of fasting in the treatment of obesity. *The Lancet*, no. ii, 1340–42.

Herman, C. P., and Mack, D. 1975. Restrained and unrestrained eating. *Journal of Personality* 43, 647–60.

Herman, C. P.; Olmsted, M. P.; and Polivy, J. In press. Obesity, externality, and susceptibility to social influence: An integrated analysis. *Journal of Personality and Social Psychology*.

Herman, C. P., and Polivy, J. 1975. Anxiety, restraint and eating behavior. *Journal of Abnormal Psychology* 84:666–72.

Herman, C. P., and Polivy, J. 1980. Restrained eating. In *Obesity*, ed. A. J. Stunkard, pp. 208–25. Philadelphia: Saunders.

Herman, C. P.; Polivy, J.; Pliner, P.; Threlkeld, J.; and Munic, D. 1978. Distractibility in dieters and nondieters: An alternative view of "externality." *Journal of Personality and Social Psychology* 36:536–48.

Herman, C. P.; Polivy, J.; and Silver, R. 1979. The effects of an observer on eating behavior: The induction of "sensible" eating. *Journal of Personality* 47:85–99.

Herman, L. S., and Iverson, M. 1968. Death during therapeutic starvation. *The Lancet*, no. i, 217.

Heyden, S.; Hames, C. G.; Bartel, A.; Cassel, J. C.; Tyroler, H. A.; and Cornoni, J. C. 1971. Weight and weight history in relation to cerebrovascular and ischemic heart disease. *Archives of Internal Medicine* 128:956–60.

References

Hibscher, J., and Herman, C. P. 1977. Obesity, dieting, and the expression of "obese" characteristics. *Journal of Comparative and Physiological Psychology* 91:374–80.

Hueneman, R. L., Shapiro, L. R., Hampton, M. C., and Mitchell, B. W. 1966. A longitudinal study of gross body composition and body conformation and their association with food and activity in a teen-age population: views of teen-age subjects on body conformation, food and activity. *American Journal of Clinical Nutrition* 18:325–38.

Jakobovits, C.; Halstead, P.; Kelley, L.; Roe, D. A.; and Young, C. M. 1977. Eating habits and nutrient intakes of college women over a thirty-year period. *Journal of the American Dietetic Association* 71:405–11.

Jameson, G., and Williams, E. 1964. *The drinking man's diet.* San Francisco: Cameron & Co.

Jung, R. T.; Shetty, P. S.; Barrand, M.; Callingham; B. A.; and James, W. P. T. 1979. Role of catecholamines in hypotensive response to dieting. *British Medical Journal* 1:12–13.

Kannel, W. B., and Gordon, T. 1974. Obesity and cardiovascular disease: The Framingham Study. In *Obesity,* ed. W. Burland, P. D. Samuel, and J. Yudkin. London: Churchill Livingstone.

Kannel, W. B.; LeBauer, E. J.; Dawber, T. R.; and McNamara, P. M. 1967. Relation of body weight to development of coronary heart disease: The Framingham study. *Circulation* 35:734–44.

Kaplan, H. I., and Kaplan, H. S. 1957. The psychosomatic concept of obesity. *Journal of Nervous and Mental Disease* 125:181–89.

Kark, R. M.; Johnson, R. E.; and Lewis, J. S. 1945. Defects of pemmican as an emergency ration for infantry troops. *War Medicine* 7:345–52.

Keesey, R. E. 1980. A set-point analysis of the regulation of body weight. In *Obesity,* ed. A. J. Stunkard, pp. 144–65. Philadelphia: Saunders.

Keys, A.; Aravanis, C.; Blackburn, H.; Van Buchem, F. S. P.; Buzina, R.; Djordjevic, B. S.; Fidanza, F.; Karvonen, M. J.; Menotti, A.; Puddu, V.; and Taylor, H. L. 1972. Coronary heart disease: Overweight and obesity as risk factors. *Annals of Internal Medicine* 77:15–27.

Keys, A.; Brozek, J.; Henschel, A.; Mickelson, O.; and Taylor, H. L. 1950. *The biology of human starvation.* 2 vols. Minneapolis: University of Minnesota Press.

Klajner, F.; Herman, C. P.; Polivy, J.; and Chhabra, R. 1981. Human obesity, dieting, and anticipatory salivation to food. *Physiology and Behavior* 27:195–98.

References

Kollar, E. J., and Atkinson, R. M. 1966. Responses of extremely obese patients to starvation. *Psychosomatic Medicine* 28:227–46.

Kollar, E. J.; Slater, G. R.; Palmer, J. O.; Docter, R. F.; and Mandell, A. J. 1964. Measurement of stress in fasting man. *Archives of General Psychiatry* 11:113–25.

Landsberg, L., and Young, J. B. 1978. Fasting, feeding and the regulation of the sympathetic nervous system. *New England Journal of Medicine* 298:1295–301.

Larsson, B.; Bjorntorp, P.; and Tibblin, G. 1981. The health consequences of moderate obesity. *International Journal of Obesity* 5:97–116.

Lavrakas, P. 1975. Female preferences for male physiques. *Journal of Research in Personality* 31:1168–76.

Leon, G. R., and Chamberlain, K. 1973a. Emotional arousal, eating patterns, and body image as differential factors associated with varying success in maintaining a weight loss. *Journal of Consulting and Clinical Psychology* 40:474–80.

Leon, G. R., and Chamberlain, K. 1973b. Comparison of daily eating habits and emotional states of overweight persons successful or unsuccessful in maintaining a weight loss. *Journal of Consulting and Clinical Psychology* 41:108–15.

Lerner, R. M. 1969a. The development of stereotyped expectancies of body build–behavior relations. *Child Development* 40:137–41.

Lerner, R. M. 1969b. Some female stereotypes of male body build–behavior relations. *Perceptual and Motor Skills* 28:363–66.

Lerner, R. M., and Gellert, E. 1969. Body build identification, preference, and aversion in children. *Developmental Psychology* 1:456–62.

Levitsky, D. A.; Faust, I.; and Glassman, M. 1976. The ingestion of food and the recovery of body weight following fasting in the naive rat. *Physiology and Behavior* 17:575–80.

McKenna, R. J. 1972. Some effects of anxiety level and food cues on the eating behavior of obese and normal subjects. *Journal of Personality and Social Psychology* 22:311–19.

Maier, R. A., and Lavrakas, P. 1981. Idealized male physique preferences. Unpublished manuscript.

Mann, G. V. 1974. The influence of obesity on health, part 1. *The New England Journal of Medicine* 291:178–85.

Marliss, E. B. 1978. Protein diets for obesity: Metabolic and clinical aspects. *Canadian Medical Association Journal* 119:1413–21.

References

Merritt, R. J.; Bistrian, B. R.; Blackburn, G. L.; and Suskind, R. L. 1980. Consequences of modified fasting in obese pediatric and adolescent patients, I: Protein-sparing modified fast. *The Journal of Pediatrics* 96:13–19.

Milich, R. S. 1975. A critical analysis of Schachter's externality theory of obesity. *Journal of Abnormal Psychology* 84:586–88.

Millman, M. 1980. *Such a pretty face: Being fat in America.* New York: W. W. Norton.

Mrosovsky, N., and Powley, T. L. 1977. Set-points for body weight and fat. *Behavioral Biology* 20:205–23.

Munro, J. F.; Maccuish, A. C.; Goodall, J. A. D.; Fraser, J.; and Duncan, L. J. P. 1970. Further experience with prolonged therapeutic starvation in gross refractory obesity. *British Medical Journal* 4:712–14.

Nisbett, R. E. 1968. Taste, deprivation, and weight determinants of eating behavior. *Journal of Personality and Social Psychology* 10:107–16.

Nisbett, R. E. 1972. Hunger, obesity, and the ventromedial hypothalamus. *Psychological Review* 79:433–53.

Olmsted, M. P. 1981. Anorexic–normal differences and predictors of concern with dieting in college women. Master's thesis Guelph University, Ontario.

Orbach, S. 1978. *Fat is a feminist issue.* London: Paddington Press.

Oster, K. A. 1980. Duplicity in a committee report on diet and coronary heart disease. *American Heart Journal* 99:409–12.

Palmer, R. L. 1979. The dietary chaos syndrome: A useful new term? *British Journal of Medical Psychology* 52:187–90.

Peck, J. W. 1978. Rats defend different body weights depending on palatability and accessibility of their food. *Journal of Comparative and Physiological Psychology* 92:555–70.

Pelkonen, R.; Nikkila, E. A.; Koskinen, S.; Penttinen, K.; and Sarna, S. 1977. Association of serum lipids and obesity with cardio-vascular mortality. *British Medical Journal* 2:1185–87.

Pliner, P. 1973. Effects of external cues on the thinking behavior of obese and normal subjects. *Journal of Abnormal Psychology* 82:233–38.

Pliner, P.; Meyer, P.; and Blankstein, K. 1974. Responsiveness to affective stimuli by obese and normal individuals. *Journal of Abnormal Psychology* 83:74–80.

Polivy, J. 1976. Perception of calories and regulation of intake in restrained and unrestrained subjects. *Addictive Behaviors* 1:237–43.

References

Polivy, J., and Herman, C. P. 1976a. The effects of alcohol on eating behavior: Disinhibition or sedation? *Addictive Behaviors* 1:121–25.

Polivy, J., and Herman, C. P. 1976b. Clinical depression and weight change: a complex relation. *Journal of Abnormal Psychology* 85:338–40.

Polivy, J., and Herman, C. P. 1976c. Effects of alcohol on eating behavior: influences of mood and perceived intoxication. *Journal of Abnormal Psychology* 85:601–6.

Polivy, J.; Herman, C. P.; and Hackett, R. 1981. Self-awareness, self-consciousness, and the inhibition of eating. Unpublished manuscript.

Polivy, J.; Herman, C. P.; Olmsted, M.; and Jazwinski, C. In press. Restraint and binge eating. In *Binge eating: theory, research and treatment*, ed. R. C. Hawkins, W. Fremouw, and P. Clement. New York: Springer Publishing Co.

Polivy, J.; Herman, C. P., and Warsh, S. 1978. Internal and external components of emotionality in restrained and unrestrained eaters. *Journal of Abnormal Psychology* 87:497–504.

Polivy, J.; Herman, C. P.; Younger, J. C.; and Erskine, B. 1979. Effects of a model on eating behavior: the induction of a restrained eating style. *Journal of Personality* 47:100–14.

Powley, T. L. 1977. The ventromedial hypothalamic syndrome, satiety, and a cephalic phase hypothesis. *Psychological Review* 84:89–126.

Pyle, R. L.; Mitchell, J. E.; and Eckert, E. D. 1981. Bulimia: A report of 34 cases. *Journal of Clinical Psychiatry* 42:60–64.

Rogers, T.; Mahoney, M. J.; Mahoney, B. K.; Straw, M. K.; and Kenigsburg, M. I. 1980. Clinical assessment of obesity: An empirical evaluation of diverse techniques. *Behavioral Assessment* 2:161–81.

Roncari, D. A. K. 1978. Personal communication.

Rooth, G., and Carlstrom, S. 1970. Therapeutic fasting. *Acta Medica Scandinavica* 187:455–463.

Rosenthal, R., and Jacobson, L. 1968. *Pygmalion in the classroom*. New York: Holt, Rinehart & Winston.

Runcie, J., and Thomson, T. J. 1970. Prolonged starvation—A dangerous procedure? *British Medical Journal* 3:432–35.

Russell, G. F. M. 1979. Bulimia nervosa: An ominous variant of anorexia nervosa. *Psychiatric Medicine* 9:429–48.

Sandhofer, F.; Diensfl, F.; Bolzano, K.; and Schwingshackl, H. 1973. Severe cardiovascular complication associated with prolonged starvation. *British Medical Journal* 1:462–63.

References

Schachter, S. 1971. Some extraordinary facts about obese humans and rats. *American Psychologist* 26:129–44.

Schachter, S. 1982. Recidivism and self-cure of smoking and obesity. *American Psychologist* 37:436–44.

Schachter, S.; Goldman, R.; and Gordon, A. 1968. Effects of fear, food deprivation, and obesity on eating. *Journal of Personality and Social Psychology* 10:107–16.

Schachter, S., and Gross, L. 1968. Air France, dormitory food, and Yom Kippur. *Journal of Personality and Social Psychology* 10:98–106.

Schachter, S., and Rodin, J. 1974. *Obese humans and rats*. Potomac, Md.: Lawrence Erlbaum Associates.

Shainess, N. 1979. The swing of the pendulum—from anorexia to obesity. *The American Journal of Psychoanalysis* 39:225–34.

Shekelle, R. B.; Shryock, A. M.; Oglesby, P.; Lepper, M.; Stamler, J.; Liu, S.; and Raynor, W.J., Jr. 1981. Diet, serum cholesterol, and death from coronary heart disease: The Western Electric study. *New England Journal of Medicine* 304:65–70.

Silverstein, B., and Kelly, E. 1982. Contradictory role expectations as a cause of eating disorders among women. Unpublished manuscript, State University of New York at Stony Brook.

Simon, R. I. 1963. Obesity as a depressive equivalent. *Journal of the American Medical Association* 183:134–36.

Sims, E. A. H. 1974. Studies in human hyperphagia. In *Treatment and management of obesity*, ed. G. Bray and J. Bethune, pp. 28–43. New York: Harper & Row.

Sjostrom, L. 1980. Fat cells and body weight. In *Obesity*, ed. A. J. Stunkard. Philadelphia: Saunders.

Slochower, J. 1976. Emotional labeling and overeating in obese and normal weight individuals. *Psychosomatic Medicine* 38:131–39.

Sorlie, P.; Gordon, T.; and Kannel, W. B. 1980. Body build and mortality —The Framingham study. *Journal of the American Medical Association* 243:1828–31.

Spencer, I. O. B. 1968. Death during therapeutic starvation for obesity. *The Lancet*, no. i, 1288–90.

Spencer, J. A., and Fremouw, W. J. 1979. Binge eating as a function of restraint and weight classification. *Journal of Abnormal Psychology* 88:262–67.

Staffieri, J. R. 1967. A study of social stereotypes of body image in children. *Journal of Personality and Social Psychology* 1:101–4.

Staffieri, J. R. 1972. Body build and behavioral expectancies in young females. *Developmental Psychology* 6:125–27.

References

Stambi, R.; Stambi, J.; Riedlinger, W.; Algera, G.; and Roberts, R. H. 1978. Weight and blood pressure—findings in hypertension screenings of one million Americans. *Journal of the American Medical Association* 240:1607–10.

Stillman, I. M., and Baker, S. S. 1967. *The doctor's quick weight loss diet.* Englewood Cliffs, N.J.: Prentice-Hall.

Stordy, B. J.; Marks, V.; Kalucy, R.S.; and Crisp, A.H. 1977. Weight gain, thermic effect of glucose and resting metabolic rate during recovery from anorexia nervosa. *American Journal of Clinical Nutrition* 30:138–46.

Stunkard, A. J. 1957. The "dieting depression." Incidence and clinical characteristics of untoward responses to weight reduction regimes. *American Journal of Medicine* 23:77–86.

Stunkard, A. J. 1972. New therapies for the eating disorders: behavior modification of obesity and anorexia nervosa. *Archives of General Psychiatry* 26:391–98.

Stunkard, A., and McLaren-Hume, M. 1959. The results of treatment for obesity—A review of the literature and report of a series. *AMA Archives of Internal Medicine* 103: 78–85.

Stunkard, A. J.; Rickels, K.; and Hesbacher, P. 1973. Fenfluramine in the treatment of obesity. *The Lancet,* no. i, 503–5.

Stunkard, A. J., and Rush, J. 1974. Dieting and depression reexamined—A critical review of reports of untoward responses during weight loss reduction for obesity. *Annals of Internal Medicine* 81:526–33.

Taller, H. 1961. *Calories don't count.* New York: Simon & Schuster.

Thomson, T. J.; Runcie, J.; and Miller, V. 1966. Treatment of obesity by total fasting for up to 249 days. *The Lancet,* no. ii, 992–96.

Woody, E. Z.; Costanzo, P. R.; Liefer, H.; and Conger, J. 1981. The effects of taste and caloric perceptions on the eating behavior of restrained and unrestrained subjects. *Cognitive Research and Therapy* 5:381–90.

Wooley, S. C.; Wooley, O. W.; and Dyrenforth, S. 1980. The case against radical interventions. *The American Journal of Clinical Nutrition* 33:465–71.

Wyden, P. 1965. *The overweight society.* New York: Morrow.

Zielinsky, J. J. 1978. Depressive symptomatology: Deviation from a personal norm. *Journal of Community Psychology* 6:163–67.

Index

Abraham, S., 67
Abramson, E. E., 178
Air Force Diet, 86
alcohol as appetite stimulant, 145–46
alienation in dieting, 166–67
alliesthesia, 44–45, 149
Alvarez, L. C., 93
American Medical Association Council on Foods and Nutrition, 87–88
amphetamines, 84
anabolic metabolism, 35, 40, 44,

56; while dieting, 166–67; difficulty of reversing, 45–46
Angel, A., 59, 70–73, 81
angina pectoris, 67
anorexia nervosa, 6, 172–76, 182; binge eating in, 169, 170, 174; as compulsion to diet, 23; dichotomous thinking in, 175; food preoccupation in, 162; force feeding as treatment for, 41–42; increase in, 101; obesity following, 175; overweight stereotypes and, 115–16; as re-

Index

anorexia nervosa *(continued)*
fusal to grow up, 121–22;
sweet preferences in, 149
anxiety: dieting and, 157–58;
hunger and, 135–36, 146–47
apomorphine, 84–85
appetite: alcohol as stimulus for,
145–46; loss of, in depression,
147–48; marijuana as stimulus
for, 145–46; stress and, 135–
36, 146–48
asceticism, symbolic aspects of,
120–23
atherosclerosis: fat cell number
and, 68; overweight and, 62
Atkins, R. C., 86
Atkinson, R. M., 81, 93
attractiveness: discipline and,
112; importance of, 109–10,
194; personality and, 110–12;
physical, of men, 107–8;
stereotyped attitudes to,
109–14

Baird, I. M., 81, 87
Ball, M. F., 92
Beck, S. B., 107
behavior therapy: to modify eating habits, 202–11; over-
weight and, 4
belladonna, 84–85
Bennett, W., 116
Berscheid, E., 111, 113
binge eating, 168–72; with ano-

rexia nervosa, 169, 170, 174;
breaking habit of, 203–4; as
consequence of dieting, 21,
170–72, 186; *see also* overeating
Bistrian, B. R., 89
Bjurlf, P., 68
Bloom, W. L., 91, 92
Boskind-Lodahl, M., 169, 170
Branch, C. H. H., 115
Bray, G. A., 58–60, 62, 69, 70,
72–74, 81, 84, 93, 94, 96
Brosin, H. W., 177
Bruch, H., 170, 174, 177,
179
bulimia, 169–74, 182
bypasses, 93–95

Cabanac, M., 148
caffeine, 163
calories: intake of, and fasting,
88–93; maintenance level of,
64–65; personal differences in
use of, 39–41, 42–43; serum
lipids and, 66
Calories Don't Count Diet, 86
Canary, J. J., 92
carbohydrates: in low-carbohydrate diets, 86–88; triglyceride
levels and, 72
Carlstrom, S., 81, 93
Casper, R. C., 170
Castro, J. H., 92
catabolism, 43

cephalic phase responses (CPRs), 164–66
Chamberlain, K., 177
CHD (coronary heart disease), 62–64
cholesterol, 71–72; gall bladder disease and, 72–73
Collins, G., 67
compulsion, 12–26; in dieting, 8, 23; see also anorexia nervosa; binge eating
coronary heart disease (CHD), 62–64
Costanzo, P., 149
CPRs (cephalic phase responses), 164–66
Cubberley, P. T., 93

death: from bypass operations, 95; from dieting, 81–82, 90; from fasting, 90; see also mortality risk
depression: appetite loss in, 147–48; with weight loss, 82, 159–60
deprivation in dieting, 13
Dermer, M., 112
diabetes, 70–71; fasting and, 88–89
diarrhea from intestinal bypasses, 94
dieting: alienation in, 166–67; anxiety and, 157–58; articles on, 102, 103, 105; binge eat-ing and, 21, 170–72, 186; books on, 103; bypasses and, 93–95; cardiovascular disease and, 66; as cause of overeating, 5–7, 21, 49, 65, 73–74, 127–28, 170–72, 178–79, 199; ce-phalic phase responses in, 164–66; compulsion in, 8, 23; dangers of, 75–99; death from, 81–82, 90; deprivation in, 13; difficulty of, 18–20; direct risks of, 80–82; distractibility in, 160–62; drugs in, 82–85; eating behavior changes and, 137–55, 188–89; eating dis-orders compared to, 185; effect on fat cells, 50–51; emo-tionality and, 157–60, 163, 182–83, 207; fad diets, 85–86; fasting in, 88–93; food preoc-cupation in, 162; hunger in, 19–20, 127–28; impact of, on body's natural regulation, 78–79; low-carbohydrate diets, 86–88; peer pressure and, 150–53, 187; prevalence of, 104, 184, 186–87; problems of, 24–25; saliva production in, 164–66; as self-control, 121–22; self-esteem and, 17–18, 123–28, 184–85; sex differ-ences in, 134–35; side effects of, 156–67, 199; stereotypes for, 25–26; stress and, 157–60,

dieting *(continued)*
162–63; sweet preference in, 148–49, 156–57; taste as factor in, 149–50; weight loss regulation and, 77–80; *see also* weight loss
diet-overeat cycle, 68–69, 73–74; *see also* binge eating
diet pills, 82–85
Diet Revolution, 86
digitalis, 84
dinitrophenol, 83
Dion, K., 111, 112
disease, overeating and, 66–69
distractibility, dieting and, 160–62
diuretics, 82, 85; with binge eating, 169
Doctor's Quick Weight Loss Diet, 86
Doell, S. R., 180
Drenick, E. J., 59, 60, 70–74, 81, 83, 84, 93
Drinking Man's Diet, 86
drugs, 43–44; in dieting, 82–85; diuretics, 82, 85, 169; laxatives, 85, 169
Duncan, G. G., 81, 91, 92
Dwyer, J. T., 104, 105, 108, 187

Eckert, E. D., 170
Ely, R. J., 178
emotionality: dieting and, 157–60, 163, 182–83; dieting difficulties and, 207; hunger as response to, 176–77, 179–80
energy, heat production and, 36
Esses, V., 145
Eurman, L. J., 115
exercise: while fasting, 91–92; metabolic adjustment and, 46; in weight control programs, 206

fad diets, 85–86
fasting, 88–93; bypasses and, 93–95; death from, 90; modified, 88–91; overweight personality and, 138; total, 91–92
fat: brown, 51–52; as burden on circulatory system, 63; difficulty of losing, 19–20; drugs to influence storage of, 83; free fatty acids (FFA), 71–72, 159, 163; heat production process and, 36; in low-carbohydrate diets, 86–87; natural weight level and, 50–51, 68; storage of, and ecological scarcity, 56; storage of, and weight changes, 34; surgical removal of, 51, 95–96
Feinstein, A. R., 83–85, 177
fenfluramine, 84
Ford, Eileen, 101
Framingham studies, 61, 67
Franklin, J. S., 171, 174
free fatty acids (FFA), 71–72; stress and, 159, 163

gall bladder disease, 72–73
Garfinkel, P. E., 101, 149, 169, 170, 175
Garner, D. M., 101, 105, 169, 170, 175
Garnett, E. S., 81, 93
Gellert, E., 117
Genuth, S. M., 92
Gilliland, I. C., 92
Glucksman, M. L., 125, 177
gluttony, 16, 64; symbolic aspects of, 120–21; see also overeating
Goldblatt, P. B., 122
Goldman, R., 178
Gordon, A., 178
Gordon, T., 61, 81
Gurin, J., 116

Hamburger, W. W., 176, 177
Harden, R. M., 92
Harrison, M. T., 92
Hawkins, R. C., 180
heart, overweight and risk to, 62–64
heat production (nonshivering thermogenesis), 36, 51
Herman, C. P., 72, 145, 170, 177, 178, 182–83
Herman, L. S., 92
Hesbacher, P., 84
Heyden, S., 67, 70
Hibscher, J., 72
Hirsch, J., 125, 177
hormone pills, 83

hormones, natural weight and, 52
Howard, A. N., 81, 87
Hueneman, R. L., 104
hunger: anxiety and, 135–36, 146–47; in dieting, 19–20, 127–28; drugs to suppress, 82, 83; emotionality and, 176–77, 179–80; getting in touch with feelings of, 199–201; hypothalamus and, 96, 131; inappropriate eating and, 178–80; lack of regulation of, 97; overweight personality and, 129–55; weight loss and, 44, 78–80
hunger suppressants, 82–84
hypertension, 63, 67, 69–70; fasting for, 88
hypothalamus, 96, 131

ideal weight: defined, 55; derivation of, 57–58; natural weight and, 59; problems of reliance on, 62; for women, 101–5; see also natural weight
International Cooperative Study of Cardiovascular Epidemiology, 63–64
Iverson, M., 92

Jakobovits, C., 104
jaw wiring, 96
Jazwinski, C., 170

jejunoileostomy, 94
Johnson, R. E., 81, 87
Jung, R. T., 81

Kannel, W. B., 61, 67, 81
Kaplan, H. I., 176, 177
Kaplan, H. S., 176, 177
Kark, R. M., 81, 87
Kelly, E., 105
Keys, A., 63, 198
Kollar, E. J., 81, 93
Kyle, L. H., 92

Landsberg, L., 81
Lavrakas, P., 107, 108
laxatives, 85; with binge eating, 169
Leon, G. R., 177
Lerner, R. M., 113, 117
lethargy from food deprivation, 44, 46
Lewis, J. S., 81, 87
lipectomy, 51, 96

McKenna, R. J., 178
McLaren-Hume, M., 81
McLear, P. M., 107
Maier, R. A., 108
Mann, G. V., 59, 63, 66, 72
marijuana as appetite stimulant, 145–46
Marliss, E. B., 81, 90
Mayer, J., 187
men: physical attractiveness of, 107–8; as restrained eaters, 134–35
Mendelson, 124
metabolism: anabolic, 35, 40, 44–46, 56, 166–67; catabolic, 43; drugs to influence, 43–44, 83; natural weight maintenance and, 35–38, 43–44, 77; personal differences in, 39–41, 42–43; thrifty, 35–36
Metropolitan Life Insurance Company, 60–61, 192
Milich, R. S., 195
Miller, V., 93
Millman, M., 113
Mitchell, J. E., 170
models, fashion, 101
Moldofsky, H., 169, 170
Moore, M. E., 122
mortality risk: heart disease and, 62; ideal weight and, 57–58; from intestinal bypasses, 95; overweight and, 60–62; from slimness, 61–62; see also death
Munro, J. F., 93

natural weight, 9, 20–21, 27–53; backlash effects and, 49; biological value of, 46–49, 76; brown fat in, 51–52; changes in level of, 52–53, 193; childhood and adult weight and, 67–68; compared to population averages, 192; control of, and peer pressure, 207–9; defined, 33; determining of personal, 197–98; diabetes and, 71; disease from ignoring, 76; dissatisfaction with, 30–32; establishment of, method for, 199–211; experimental work on, 27–30, 131–32; fat cells in determination of, 50–51, 68; health and, 55–56, 76; hormones and, 52; hypertension and, 70; ideal weight and, 59; individual differences in, 33–34; lethargy as defense for, 44, 46; mechanisms for maintaining, 34–38, 117; metabolism as defense for, 35–38, 43–44, 77; overweight personality and, 135–55; range differences in, 42, 193; regulation of, and weight loss, 77–80, 125; sweet craving as defense for, 44–45; in treatment of anorexia nervosa, 42

neurosis, dieting and, 127

Nisbett, Richard, 5, 131–32, 136, 149

nonshivering thermogenesis, 36, 51

Nordsieck, M., 67

obesity: adult onset vs. juvenile onset, 195; after anorexia nervosa, 175; attractiveness and, 113; coronary heart disease and, 63; defined, 59; diabetes and, 71; drugs for treatment of, 83–85; fasting for, 91–92; gall bladder disease and, 73; health effects of, 59–60; hypertension and, 70; hypothalamus and, 131; natural weight and, 137; psychosomatic theory of, 176; serum lipids and, 71–72; stereotypes of, 114–20; surgical solutions for, 51, 93–96; see also overweight

Olmsted, M. P., 108, 170

Orbach, S., 106, 113, 122, 177, 180, 181

overeating: defined, 65; diabetes and, 71; dieting as cause of, 5–9, 21, 49, 65, 73–74, 127–28, 170–72, 178–79, 199; diet-overeat cycle, 68–69, 73–74; disease and, 66–69; gluttony, 16, 64, 120–21; hunger suppressants for, 82, 83; overweight and, 64–66; after rapid weight loss, 80; see also binge eating; obesity

overweight: assumptions on causes of, 3–4; coronary heart disease (CHD) and, 62–64; dieting as cause of, 5–7; dangers of, 57–74; defined, 59; diabe-

Index

overweight *(continued)*
 tes and, 70–71; experiments to
 encourage, 29–30; extraneous
 stimuli and, 4–5; gall bladder
 disease and, 72–73; health
 hazards of, 16; hypertension
 and, 69–70; mortality risk and,
 60–62; overeating and, 64–66;
 personality and, 114–20, 129–
 55; physical attractiveness
 and, 113–14; scarce ecology
 and, 56–57; self-esteem and,
 17, 123–28; serum lipids and,
 71–72; sex differences in,
 105–7; stereotyped attitudes
 toward, 15–16, 17, 74, 101,
 113–20; stress and, 157–60; as
 unacceptable condition, 13–
 15; *see also* obesity

Palmer, R. L., 169
Parsons, R. L., 81, 87
peer pressure: dieting and, 150–
 53, 187; and natural weight
 control, 207–9; for slimness,
 100–7, 194
Pelkonen, R., 62
personality: attractiveness and,
 110–12; fat vs. thin, 114–20;
 overweight, 114–20, 129–55
physicians' reactions to overweight patients, 74, 93
Playboy, 101–2, 105
Playgirl, 105

Pliner, P., 158, 161–62
Polivy, J., 104, 145, 170, 177,
 178, 182, 183
Polster, S. A., 93
potassium, loss of, in fasting, 88–
 90, 93
Powley, T., 164
protein: fasting and, 88, 89; in
 low-carbohydrate diets, 86–87
psychological reasons for weight
 gain, 180–81
psychological symptoms of
 weight loss, 28
Pyle, R. L., 170

refeeding: after fasting, 90; as
 treatment for anorexia ner-
 vosa, 42
Restrained eating, 129–67; *see
 also* dieting
Restraint Scale, 132–34, 135,
 143, 149
Rickels, K., 84
Rodin, J., 131, 178
Rogers, T., 72
Roncari, D. A. K., 59–60, 70–73,
 81
Rooth, G., 81, 93
Runcie, J., 93
Rush, J., 92
Russell, G. F. M., 169, 170

saliva, production of, while dieting, 164–66

Index

Sandhofer, F., 93

satiety: cues for, 78–80; getting in touch with feelings of, 199–201; inappropriate eating and, 178–80; lack of regulation of, 97, 127–28; overweight personality and, 129–55

Schachter, S., 4–5, 129, 135–38, 142, 143, 146, 157, 160, 161, 178, 186, 195

Schulman, C. L., 93

Schwartz, D., 101

self-control, 17; in anorexia nervosa, 172–74; depression and, 148; weight loss and, 180

self-denial, 17

self-discipline: attractiveness and, 112; in dieting, 121–22

self-esteem, 17–18; slimness and, 123–28, 184–85

serum lipids: calorie intake and, 66; overweight and, 71–72

sexuality: weight gain and, 180–81; weight loss and, 126, 175

Sherman, M., 89

Silverstein, B., 105

Simon, R. I., 177

slimness: asceticism and, 121; desirability of, 14–15, 114–19; as female ideal, 101–5; as indulgence, 121–22; as male ideal, 108; mortality risk in, 61–62; personality and, 114–

20; self-esteem and, 123–28, 184–85; sex differences in desire for, 105–7, 108; social pressures for, 100–7, 194; stereotyped attitudes toward, 15, 17, 21–22, 101; success and, 122

Slochower, J., 178

Sorlie, P., 61

spas, 102–3

Spencer, I. O. B., 93

Staffieri, J. R., 113, 117

Stambi, R., 69

Stillman, I. M., 86

stomach, surgery to close off part of, 96

stress: appetite effects of, 135–36, 146–48; dieting and, 157–60, 162–63; free fatty acids and, 159, 163

strokes, weight gain and, 67

Stunkard, A. J., 81, 84, 92, 122, 124, 196

success, slimness and, 122

surgery: bypass operations, 93–95; to remove fat, 51, 95–96

sweets: aversive reaction to, 44–45; dieters' responses to, 148–49, 156–57

Taller, H., 86

Thiel, D., 112

Thompson, M., 101

Thompson, T. J., 93
triglycerides, 71–72

undereating, see dieting

Veterans Administration, 71
vomiting: with binge eating, 169;
for weight control, 23

Walster, Elaine, 111, 113
Ward-Hull, C. I., 107
Warsh, S., 178
water in daily weight fluctuation,
34
weight, distribution of, in population, 191–92
weight gain: diabetes and, 71;
gall bladder disease and, 73;
hypertension and, 70; natural
defenses against, 37–38;
psychological reasons for,
180–81; strokes and, 67; as
unnatural development, 66–
67, 195
weight loss: cultural emphasis on,
116–19; depression with, 82,
159–60; difficulty of, 18–20,
193; direct risks of, 80–82; experiment to encourage, 27–29;
"good" vs. "bad," 76–77; hunger and, 44, 78–80; hypertension and, 70; natural defenses
against, 37–38; negative
effects of, 28–29; psychological symptoms of, 28; regulation of natural weight and,
77–80; self-control and, 180;
self-esteem and, 123–28, 184–
85; serum lipids and, 72; sexuality and, 126, 175; see also
dieting
will power as personality characteristic, 116–19
women: binge eating by, 168–70;
as restrained eaters, 134–35;
social pressures for slimness of,
100–7, 187
Woody, E., 149
Wooley, O. W., 95
Wooley, S. C., 95
Wunderlich, R. A., 178
Wyden, P., 104

Young, J. B., 81

Zielinsky, J. J., 177